Managing Money for General Practitioners

SECOND EDITION

Managing Money for General Practitioners

SECOND EDITION

Edited by

Mike Gilbert

Partner
RMT Accountants & Business Advisors
Newcastle upon Tyne

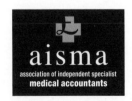

Radcliffe Publishing
Oxford • New York

Radcliffe Publishing Ltd
18 Marcham Road
Abingdon
Oxon OX14 1AA
United Kingdom

www.radcliffe-oxford.com

Electronic catalogue and worldwide online ordering facility.

British Library Cataloguing in Publication Data

A catalogue record for this book is available from the British Library.

ISBN-13: 978 184619 265 4

Typeset by Pindar New Zealand (Egan Reid), Auckland, New Zealand
Printed and bound by TJ International, Padstow, Cornwall, UK

Contents

Preface to the second edition

The running of a medical practice in the 21st century has all the trimmings of running a business. Instead of a move towards a salaried profession, which was envisaged 12 years ago, in reality the opposite has occurred, with GPs more than ever in control of their own financial destiny. Now that the new contract has bedded down, it is timely to take a fresh look at general practice finance.

This book is meant to be an essential guide to the complexities of practice finances and the running of a successful practice for both GPs and practice managers. The format is intended to be easy to use, and throughout there are worked examples and tables which can be lifted and applied to the reader's own circumstances. If this book doesn't help GPs and practice managers in their own practices then we have failed to achieve our purpose.

I am grateful to members of the Association of Independent Specialist Medical Accountants (AISMA) executive who have so ably contributed to this book. Without their assistance this book would not have been possible.

To help keep this book up to date why not contact your nearest AISMA member and ask to be put on their mailing list to receive the AISMA quarterly newsletter? They may even provide you with a binder to put them in! By keeping the newsletters close to this book you will be able to capture all future changes in the world of medical finance. You will find the list of AISMA members at the AISMA website, www.aisma.org.uk.

You might also find helpful information to assist you with practice finance.

Michael Gilbert
October 2008

About the editor

Michael Gilbert is a chartered accountant who has specialised in the financial accountancy and taxation of members of the medical profession for over 25 years. He is accepted as a leading authority on the subject and is in considerable demand as a lecturer to doctors and practice managers alike, and for contributions to the medical press.

Michael also writes and comments extensively for medical journals. He is the author of the AISMA publication *The Medical Practitioner's Handbook*, and is currently responsible for the production of the quarterly AISMA newsletter.

Michael set up the specialist medical division in RMT accountants and business advisors in Newcastle upon Tyne in 1991, and they currently act for over 135 medical practices. RMT is responsible for the AISMA annual survey into the accounts of GPs and the subsequent production of national benchmarking profiles. Michael was a founder member of AISMA and from 1997 to 2002 was Chairman of the Association.

Contributors

All of the following contributors are executive members of the committee of the Association of Independent Specialist Medical Accountants (AISMA) in the UK.

Sue Beaton is a director of Coveney Nicholls in Reigate and heads up its medical division. She drafted Chapter 8 of the book.

Luke Bennett is a partner of Winter Rule in Cornwall and in charge of their healthcare clients. He drafted Chapter 6 of the book and assisted with Chapter 15.

David Clough is a partner in the accounting firm of Charles Rippin and Turner in North London and is currently the Chairman of AISMA. He drafted Chapters 1 and 14 of the book.

Liz Densley is a partner in the accounting firm of Honey Barrett in Eastbourne and Bexhill on Sea and is currently the Secretary of AISMA. She drafted Chapter 13 of the book.

Chris Howe is a director in the accounting firm Foxley Kingham in Luton, and drafted Chapter 12 of the book.

Andrew Johnson is a partner in the accounting firm of Creers in York. He drafted Chapter 15 of the book.

Bob Senior is a director of the national accounting firm Tenon in its Eastleigh office and is currently the Vice Chairman of AISMA. He drafted Chapter 9 of the book.

Kevin Walker is an independent financial advisor and director of RMT Financial Management Limited in Newcastle upon Tyne. He assisted the editor in the drafting of Chapter 11 of the book.

Deborah Wood is the specialist medical partner of Moore & Smalley in Blackpool, Preston and Fleetwood, and is a former President of the North West Society of Chartered Accountants. She drafted Chapters 5 and 10 of the book, and acknowledges the assistance of Ross Mathieson at the NHS Pensions Agency, Tom Young at the Inland Revenue, and David Walker, the tax consultant at Moore and Smalley.

Acknowledgements

The editor acknowledges the valuable and professional contribution made by Dr Simon Cartwright of Oxford through the auspices of his book, *Contract 2003: A GP's Guide to Earning the Most* (Butterworth-Heinemann; 2003). His understanding of the issues relating to the running of a medical practice as a business is second to none, and it was a pleasure working with him.

Michael Gilbert
October 2008

Introduction

More than ever, it is inappropriate to expect high earnings just for working hard as a good doctor. Nor is it appropriate to expect high earnings for operating systems that suited the old contract. The most financially successful medical practices must be prepared for change, willing to embrace new opportunities and be competent to set up the right systems. Those general practitioners earning the highest incomes in medical practice make financial wealth a high priority. However, it is recognised that GPs have different priorities – many put patient care and quality of life higher up the priority ladder than finance. At the end of the day, the pursuit of higher income is a decision for the partners, and will be reached after much soul searching. The agreement among the partners of this balance between lifestyle, money and patient care is the key to a stable practice. When partners disagree about this balance, dispute inevitably occurs and the practice suffers.

Under the old contract, higher earners tended to have large list sizes, rigorously claimed all fees and allowances they were entitled to, maximised outside earnings and were normally the first movers into government-led initiatives that brought financial inducements. The new contract opens up different opportunities for income generation, although many of the old principles still apply. It has placed high income within the sights of many more practices, and gives practices more control over how to manage their profitability without, of course, compromising patient medical care. Hence the need for a book about GP finance.

There are many people who assume that because GPs are paid mainly from the public purse their incomes must be broadly similar, so that the 'average' earnings will not be far from either the top or the bottom earners. The AISMA survey into the earnings of GPs in 2007 demonstrates that this is not the case at all. In a survey of 1,836 practices representing over 18% of all practices in the UK, the following range of earnings was identified. The figures relate to the average profit share of a full-time equivalent partner in the practice.

Earnings per annum	Number of practices	%
Under £80,000	105	6
£81,000 to £100,000	331	18
£101,000 to £120,000	501	27
£121,000 to £150,000	528	29
£151,000+	371	20
Total	1,836	100

Given the width of the above range it is reasonable to assume that there is a need for a guide to medical finance.

However, a guide can only be just that, and even the best professional advice available is not enough to ensure that GPs maximise their incomes. Much has to be done 'inside' the practice, and this has to be partner led. It is up to the equity partners to ensure that the appropriate skills are available within the practice staff team, particularly in terms of practice management and accounting procedures. GPs can, of course, delegate, but they can never abdicate. Within every practice there must be someone who has a detailed knowledge of the contract. Much of the income generated by the new contract is calculated automatically by the primary care trust (PCT) using sophisticated computer technology, but this does not mean that errors cannot be made. On the contrary, it is the experience of the contributors to this book that errors often occur and practices do not always receive everything to which they are entitled.

It follows that someone in every practice must check in detail the monthly schedules provided by the PCTs and confirm their accuracy to the GP partners. The documentation provided varies between PCTs. As a simple example, is the practice being paid for the correct number of points achieved under the Quality and Outcomes Framework? Other items that need attention include list size for the calculation of the global lump sum, the payment for agreed enhanced services and the application of nationally agreed uplifts. For practices that provide personal medical services, it is essential to check the contract sum regularly, particularly when there are variations, and certainly from one year to the next.

The new contract still embraces items that need to be claimed for on a regular basis, such as PCT board member or other salaries, locum fees for PCT meetings, flu vaccinations, drugs and other PCT-administered income. All too often PCTs 'forget' to make payments to which practices are entitled, or they make payments very late indeed. The moral of the story is that PCT accounting is by no means perfect, and GPs must ensure that they have strong claiming and checking systems in their own practices so that they can be confident that nothing is missed.

All this means that, in the modern world, GPs, although delegating many of their management and administration functions to practice managers and other highly qualified staff, must remain aware of the manner in which they are paid, how their income is taxed, how their tax will be settled and the numerous financial problems that can arise in partnerships. The contents of this book have been arrived at with this in mind, so that GPs and practice managers alike will have a practical guide to the financial issues affecting medical practice.

While every effort has been made during the preparation of this book to ensure that information is as up to date as possible, readers should bear in mind that contract pricing, sources of income, tax rates and interest rates can change at relatively short notice. In particular, the rate of change to medical practice finance in the past few years has been enormous. Consequently, the most up-to-date advice should always be sought when making any decisions based on the information given in this book.

CHAPTER 1

The legal framework of a medical practice

The National Health Service (NHS) was born in 1948. Since then there have been many changes, with a major reorganisation in 1990. A new general practitioner (GP) contract was introduced and, together with earlier changes from 1966, has been the basis of a medical practice's income and its working practice. Radical proposals were introduced on 1 April 2004 based on protracted negotiations from October 2001, which were based on findings from a survey of GPs. The proposals endeavoured to rectify many of the findings brought to light, such as low morale, high workloads, and dissatisfaction with pay and conditions.

The Department of Health (DoH) was set up to support the government to improve healthcare, set standards and secure resources to deliver services to the country. To help achieve their aims, strategic health authorities (SHAs) were set up in April 2002.

SHAs have the role of developing strategies for the NHS and ensuring that local NHS organisations deliver services well. To achieve this, primary care trusts (PCTs) were created, with the responsibility of managing healthcare in a local area.

PCTs are statutory bodies that receive 75% of the NHS budget, and liaise with local authorities and other agencies to provide health needs at the primary and secondary levels. Being local, their role is to assess local needs based on their knowledge, and plan accordingly. PCTs have autonomy and much responsibility. Their powers are far reaching and include commissioning of services and purchase of property.

Primary care is provided by GPs, dentists, opticians, pharmacists and, more recently, walk-in centres, which provide instant access to advice and treatment. Secondary care is provided through acute, ambulance, care and mental health trusts. Most patients will be referred to secondary care by their GP, although in certain situations GPs can provide secondary care, e.g. counselling.

Figure 1.1 summarises all of the above.

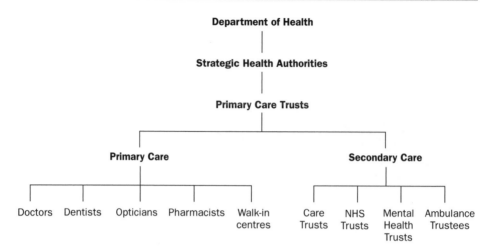

Figure 1.1 The organisation of the health service.

THE MEDICAL PRACTICE

General practitioners provide primary care, with the power to refer to secondary care. Their role is to provide healthcare in a designated local area and provide basic advice and treatment. They can also provide education to encourage preventative medicine, give vaccinations and carry out simple surgical operations.

To fund the practice, GPs receive income from the PCT, the amount depending on whether they provide general medical services (GMS) or personal medical services (PMS). Funding is discussed in Chapter 5. Changes to the GMS contract were introduced in April 2004, and the financial bible is now the Statement of Financial Entitlements (SFE), which replaces the familiar 'Red Book' that has adorned GPs' bookshelves for over 40 years. The SFE sets out the guidance relating to payments made by a PCT to a contractor under a GMS contract. Copies of the document are available from the DoH website www.dh.gov.uk.

GENERAL PRACTITIONER STATUS

GPs are unique as independent contractors to the NHS. GPs are treated as self-employed individuals who pay their own tax and national insurance liabilities. They are responsible for organising and paying for their surgery, staff and other overheads. However, as far as their income is concerned, they have limited control and, as will be seen later in this book, the generation of income is on a very different footing to that of other self-employed professionals.

Although generally self-employed, the GP is entitled to be a member of the NHS Pension Scheme – an occupational scheme for employees. Full details of this scheme are discussed in Chapter 10, but suffice to say at this stage that although GPs pay between 5% and 8.5% of their superannuable earnings into their scheme, the employer, i.e. the PCT, is responsible for a further 14%. Other self-employed persons do not have this attractive advantage.

Great care must be taken to ensure that the correct status is awarded to a doctor. The recent changes to both PMS and GMS contracts have encouraged many doctors to become salaried partners or doctors. This category of doctor is rarely self-employed, and professional advice should be sought to ensure that the GP obtains the status best suited to their individual circumstances.

CHAPTER 2

The structure of medical practice

The business structure of general practice has been run along traditional lines since the inception of the NHS in 1948. Practices have been run by the partners who have actually performed most of the clinical work. This structure was encouraged by the old 'Red Book' rules, particularly the calculation of the basic practice allowance and the restriction on GP Principal numbers imposed by the Medical Practices Committee. Thus, prior to the new contract only the minority of the workforce was made up of salaried doctors, registrars, assistants or locums.

The new contract changes all this, and many commentators refer to the key issue of the new contract as being skills-mix. It is now entirely up to individual practices how they structure both the business management and medical workforce within their walls. Indeed, it is no longer necessary to replace a retiring partner with an identical substitute in order to maintain practice income. It is financially favourable to restrict the number of profit-sharing partners to maximise individual shares and to employ salaried doctors or other healthcare individuals to help provide medical care.

In the current climate, when an existing partner retires the continuing partners can take the opportunity to consider whether the outgoing partner should be replaced by a different healthcare professional who will bring alternative skills to the practice. They also look to achieve list sizes that provide for optimum use of existing partners. Practices are therefore striving to achieve the ideal practice structure with a view to maximising profits. The new contract has made medical practice more of a business than a salaried service, with the partners effectively acting as shareholders. While the common mission statement of a practice might be 'to provide the highest quality of medical care', there will always be the tacit aim of maximising profit alongside. It is no longer good enough simply to expect money to flow in for being a good doctor, as such a policy always produces a mediocre financial reward. To achieve above-average rewards, GPs have to be prepared for change, willing to embrace new opportunities and positive in setting up the right systems.

The ideal structure of the practice will be dictated by several factors, such as:

- the availability of doctors in the area
- the partners' preferences for providing management/specialisation/out of hours
- the skills of other employed staff
- the management culture
- opportunities for work outside the practice
- competition with other local providers
- the demographics of the local population.

Opportunities to change a practice's structure may occur only when an existing partner retires or resigns. In the meantime, practices need to consider changing the practice list size in order to change the balance of staff and partners. Alternatively, practices can consider merging or splitting partnerships, particularly when recruitment of partners is a major difficulty.

There are, of course, other issues that need to be considered when attempting to formulate the ideal practice structure. These include the following.

- Should the practice diversify into non-GMS/PMS activities?
- Should the practice appoint a specialist firm of accountants, or indeed a management consultant?
- Should the practice change its information technology systems to ensure that the system is capable of recording quality data, retrieving quality data and dealing with electronic claims?

Given that the ideal practice structure is geared to maximise earnings, it is worth knowing the common features of both high and low earners. In conducting their annual survey into the accounts of their GP clients, Association of Independent Specialist Medical Accountants (AISMA) members have been able to identify, on a regular basis, the features that determine whether practices are high earners or low earners. High earners have the following features:

- stable partnership (low turnover of partners)
- partners work as a team, trust each other, plan ahead and meet regularly
- top-rate databases on patients and treatments
- partners have similar philosophies in terms of the dichotomy between money and patient care
- proactive rather than reactive teams
- good managers of time
- well-organised GPs with strong staff teams and good skills-mix among them
- GPs who delegate well to nurses, health visitors, etc.
- GPs who work long hours, have low deputising costs and a high level of non-NHS earnings
- GPs with very high list sizes (normally single-handed GPs)
- GPs who have the ability to dispense

- PMS GPs who have taken advantage of growth funding and freed up time to perform more lucrative tasks
- GPs who are heavily involved with their primary care organisation (PCO)
- GPs with the most competent and skilled practice managers and specialist accountants
- GPs who were early fundholders.

In fact, these features could well represent a guide to those GPs earning the most. Practices should score themselves out of 10 for each of the 15 items above – a total of 125 or more means a good performance, a score of 100-plus is average, and a score of less than 100 means that practices have work to do *on* the practice, not *in* the practice, to increase earnings significantly.

The features of the low-earning practices who, under the new contract, could expect financial disaster to befall are:

- practices involved in partnership disputes
- GPs with inadequate resources, such as staff, equipment and space (such GPs often have the wrong staff-mix or have a loyal contingent of staff who have been promoted over the years but do not necessarily have the relevant skills)
- badly organised practices that typically have an excessive number of patients; poor internal control systems are a feature of such practices
- GPs who are bad managers of time
- GPs who work as individuals and not as a team, who gave little or no thought to fundholding or an early entrance into PMS
- new practices with low list sizes
- practices in very deprived areas
- GPs who value 'time off' way over and above money, who incur very high deputising costs and have a low non-NHS income
- GPs without the necessary data available on their patients, either through neglect or through poor skills-mix among the staff.

Practices should determine how many of the above apply to them. Seven or more can spell financial disaster, four or more may require a new and determined approach, and one to three probably require some tinkering to be done.

When considering the ideal practice structure, many practices find it difficult to get started. Perhaps the best approach is to hold an 'away day', possibly facilitated by a consultant or the practice accountant. The ultimate objective of the away day is to produce a plan, probably in writing. To achieve this, the partners and any others present should base the discussion on answering and debating the key questions in the table below honestly.

Six key questions	Information to consider
1 What do we want to do?	The personal aspirations of the partners regarding healthcare, earnings, general goals and environment
2 What have we done in the past?	A critical analysis of current and past performance
3 What must we do well to succeed?	The key success factors
4 What could we do?	The strengths and weaknesses in terms of resources – skills, staffing, space, finance, etc.
5 What might we do?	The opportunities and threats in a changing environment
6 What should we do?	The identification and evaluation of a range of options arising from questions (1) to (5)

If the away-day debate is lively, honest and focused, the practice will be able to come up with a plan to achieve the ideal practice structure. The plan, which should be in written form, might include:

- practice objective and philosophy
- quality of healthcare
- practice profile and list size
- patient services
- organisation charge and lines of authority
- partner roles
- practice staff team
- delegated responsibility
- practice premises
- prescribing and referral patterns
- partnership succession
- technology and information systems
- profit and cash forecasts
- outside appointments
- key success factors.

It should be noted that partner roles are included in the above plan. In an ideal practice, all partners should share the feeling of responsibility for income generation. In this respect there are specific roles that are best divided up among the partners, who in turn report to the partnership on a regular basis. It is important that tasks are allocated to the best person for each job. While some of the tasks can be delegated to the practice manager, they should not be abdicated, and partners should be given protected time for management. This enables the job to be done more effectively, the benefit of which almost invariably outweighs the cost to the practice.

With the new contract in mind, the specific roles to be allocated might be as follows:

- managing or senior partner responsible for the coordination of the various

partner roles and the development and implementation of partnership strategy
- finance and accounts
- personnel and training
- premises
- clinical quality
- organisational quality
- additional services
- enhanced services
- prescribing and dispensing
- primary healthcare team (PCO liaison)
- private work.

Note that the clinical quality areas will probably be divided up among the partners. Thus, an organisation chart of a typical four-partnered practice might

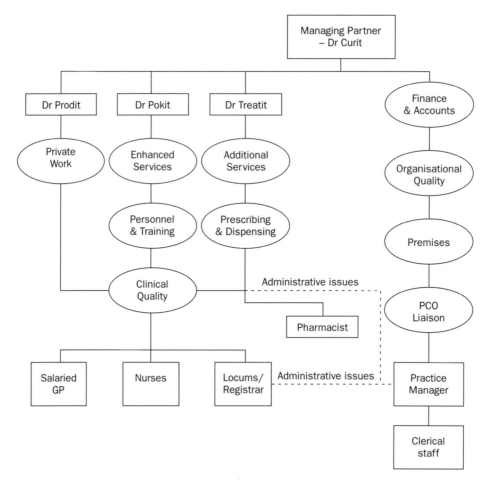

Figure 2.1 The organisation chart of a typical four-partnered practice.

look like the one in Figure 2.1. It will be noted that the practice manager should report directly to the managing or senior partner, but in practice he or she will have some obligations to the other partners and, indeed, to the other health professionals.

Finally, the role of the practice manager is crucial to the ideal practice structure. The qualifications of practice managers in the UK vary enormously. Some are promoted receptionists and others are recruited with specific professional or management qualifications. The responsibilities given to practice managers also vary enormously from practice to practice. GPs often struggle to determine exactly what to delegate and what to retain for themselves. The box below gives suggestions for the general duties and responsibilities of a modern-day practice manager which could well form the basis of an appropriate job specification.

Suggested general duties and responsibilities of a modern-day practice manager:

Administration
- Employ locums.
- Organise rotas – holidays and out of hours (if not opted out).
- Assist with teaching medical students.
- Prepare and control partnership contracts.
- Arrange, chair and minute practice meetings.
- Control over legal matters.
- Arrange professional indemnity cover and group locum insurance.

Quality assurance
- Responsibility for patient services and implementing service standards.
- Set up quality improvement monitoring systems and complaints procedures.
- Establish patient charter and ensure full confidentiality for patients.
- Ensure clinics are well organised.
- Supervise appointment system.
- Set up ways to improve patient participation.
- Produce patient leaflet or brochure.
- Produce annual reports and be responsible for audits.
- Assist with practice policy generally, and help to set up systems.

Human resources
- Responsibility for all practice staff and their work environment and welfare.
- Select and recruit practice staff. Discipline and dismiss staff when necessary.

- Be aware of current employment legislation.
- Responsibility for staff contracts, job descriptions, training needs and appraisals.
- Organise welcome packs and all staff and locums.
- Produce staff development plans.
- Responsibility for staff training, staff meetings and external courses.
- Negotiate staff budgets and control over same.
- Responsibility for health and safety policy.
- Establish an effective primary healthcare team.
- Develop role of nurse practitioners, including training issues.

Finance

- Responsibility for maintaining accounting records and management information.
- Responsibility for salary and PAYE/national insurance contributions (NIC) records.
- Monitor all claims and payments.
- Assist with profit improvement by exploring areas for increasing income or reducing costs.
- Responsibility for insurance, pension schemes, etc.
- Approve invoices for payment.
- Liaise with bankers and practice accountant.

Premises

- Responsibility for all building projects.
- Responsibility for maintenance contracts and general upkeep.
- Responsibility for housekeeping and cleaners.

Strategy

- Review and update practice vision statement.
- Facilitate production of business plans.
- Facilitate the production of bids for additional funding.
- Monitor progress against business plans and visions.
- Assist the practice in the wider community.
- Take lead in 'Investor in People' issues.

Information technology

- Assist with purchase of appropriate information systems (in liaison with PCO).
- Ensure practice keeps up to date with technological issues.
- Responsibility for library.
- Operate 'links' systems.
- Ensure practice is fully compliant with latest NHS recommendations.

Interface

- Build and maintain good working relationship with PCO, hospitals, community agencies, local medical committee (LMC), other GP practices, pharmacists, etc.
- Represent practice at meetings and seminars in the region.
- With the partners, produce own personal development plan, including training.
- Present professional image and always promote the practice.
- Share skills and expertise with others.

There is no doubt that the nature of medical practice is changing. GPs must embrace change and move forward. Practice-based commissioning is another issue that cannot be ignored, whether by practice or by locality. Practices either get on and do the job or the threat of alternative providers in the primary care market becomes a very real possibility, particularly among the smaller practices who find it more difficult to cope.

CHAPTER 3

Partnership agreements

In new general medical services, the practice is the GMS or PMS contractor. This can be:

- an individual medical practitioner
- two or more individuals practising in partnership, at least one of whom must be a medical practitioner
- certain types of companies limited by shares, where at least one share in the company is legally and beneficially owned by a medical practitioner.

The most common form of contractor remains a group of individuals practising in partnership. However, it is becoming more common for partnerships to include not only medical practitioners but also practice managers, nurses, dentists, consultants, pharmacists or other allied health professionals.

In the absence of a partnership agreement there is a 'partnership at will', which means that relations between partners are governed by the Partnership Act 1890. This is an unstable business relationship, as the partnership can be dissolved at any time with the following consequences.

- A notice may be served by any one partner on the others without their prior knowledge or consent, which takes immediate effect, and no reason need be given to justify it.
- The notice may result in the forced sale of all partnership assets (including surgery premises) and the redundancy of all staff – this creates the potential to incur considerable financial loss.
- Following dissolution, some of the partners may wish to set up in practice again, but there is no guarantee that they will be able to obtain a new GMS or PMS contract.
- There is no restrictive covenant.

It therefore follows that the positive reasons for having a partnership agreement are:

- to reduce the risk of contentious and expensive disputes

- to protect the financial interest of each partner
- to satisfy the interest of primary care organisations
- to enable GPs to write their own rules
- to deal effectively with the appointment and retirement of partners.

Given that partners are jointly and severally liable for each other's actions and the obligations of the practice as a whole, a well-drafted partnership agreement is almost a necessity in ensuring that the partners are provided with security and stability.

When drawing up a partnership agreement or amending an existing agreement, practices should seek specialist legal, accountancy and tax advice. Further partnership advice may also be obtained from the LMC or so far as concerns British Medical Association (BMA) members, from their local BMA office.

Specialist lawyers drafting partnership agreements on behalf of medical practices tend to suggest the following contents and framework.

- Parties to the agreement.
- Definitions of terms used in the agreement.
- Interpretations.
- Recitals (including nature of business, GMS or PMS and whether an NHS body).
- Consideration and covenant.
- Nature of partnership and place of business.
- Commencement date and duration of the partnership.
- Partnership capital and surgery premises.
- *Rights of occupation in surgery premises.*
- The requirement to set up a 'sinking fund' in respect of leasehold premises.
- Amount of capital to be maintained by each partner.
- Loans and advances to the partnership.
- Rate, if any, of interest payable on fixed capital or loans and advances.
- The practice accountants, solicitors and bankers.
- Partnership bank accounts and cheque signatories.
- The accounting date and details of what constitutes the practice accounts.
- *Valuations (including the exclusion of goodwill).*
- *The constitution of partnership income and individual income, including directed payments and reimbursements, and prior shares of 'profit'.*
- Legacies and gifts.
- *The expenses of the partnership.*
- *The individual expenses of the partners and requirement to complete in a timely fashion.*
- *The allocation and treatment of superannuation contributions.*
- Shares of profits and losses.
- Absences and locums, including holidays, education, illness, maternity, paternity, adoption, compassionate leave, service in armed forces and jury service.

- Partners' obligations to each other.
- *Quality and Outcomes Framework.*
- *Financial arrangements surrounding out-of-hours activities.*
- Restrictions on actions of partners.
- Insurance and indemnity.
- Patients.
- Decision making.
- Mediation.
- Arbitration.
- *Period of mutual assessment.*
- Voluntary retirement.
- Compulsory retirement.
- Fitness to practise.
- The effect of retirement, including financial entitlements.
- Restrictions on retired partner.
- Acquisition and sale of shares in the partnership capital.
- Purchase of a share of the partnership capital on the retirement or death of a partner.
- Specific responsibilities, including the nominated partner for partnership taxation matters and the responsibilities thereof, the nominated person responsible for compliance with the Data Protection Act 1998, etc.
- Signature of partnership documents and the binding of all partners to the contract with the primary care trust.
- Notices.
- Further assurance.
- Costs.
- Certificate of value.

Much of the above states the obvious and does not require any further comment at this stage. However, some of the contents have major financial consequences, particularly following the introduction of the new contract; these items are italicised above for further consideration.

On admitting a new partner, a new partnership agreement or deed of variation to an existing agreement is required, and must be signed before the first day of any period of mutual assessment to avoid the possibility of a 'partnership at will' arising. A well-drafted agreement will allow for a period of mutual assessment, allowing either the existing partners or the new partner to give notice if either side does not wish to continue the arrangement, while leaving the original partnership agreement intact.

Ownership of surgery premises can invariably be a thorny issue, and there are differing views relating to the basis of valuation. It is essential that the partners agree the basis at the outset and record it clearly in the partnership agreement. They should also agree upon what happens to incoming and outgoing partners. It is not essential that all partners should be owners of the premises. Indeed, ownership of the premises can be in different shares to the normal profit-sharing arrangements, and there is still no need to use a separate business vehicle. However, non-property-owning partners should be granted a licence to occupy for the duration of the medical partnership by the property-owning partners.

Under the new contract it is now more important than ever for the partners to agree precisely what constitutes partnership income and what constitutes either private income or a prior share of partnership profit. This will more than likely require the partners to be absolutely clear about what is and what is not partnership *time*. In this context, GPs should be aware that under GMS2 seniority payments, returners scheme payments and golden hello scheme payments have to be paid directly to the partner concerned. Moreover, if the practice decides to opt out of the provision of out-of-hours services, the agreement may allow for an individual partner to perform such work and retain the income personally, provided of course that the affairs of the practice are not harmed in any way. Finally, the partners should agree on how to apportion quality aspiration and achievement payments. Normally, this would be on a straight apportionment basis, which means an end-year apportionment in the same proportion as the partnership share, reduced by the number of days missing from the full year in question.

In a similar way, the partners should agree on what expenses are to be met by the partnership, what expenses are to be met personally and what partnership expenses are to be prior charged to individual partners. The more common items to consider in this regard are spouses' salaries, home and mobile telephones, courses and conferences, locum insurance, subscriptions and personal account-ancy fees. Practices are advised that strictness is not necessarily the best course, as partners have an insurable interest in one another – being reasonable with one another inevitably results in the most appropriate solution.

The calculation of superannuation contributions and superannuable income since 1 April 2004 is based on the taxable income of each and every individual GP after eliminating the 'profit' relating to non-NHS work. Thus, the taxable income can include profit share, private income and prior shares of profit for each GP, together with their attributable share of partnership expenses, personal expenses and prior charges of profit. It follows therefore that the contributions of GPs in a practice will almost certainly not be in normal profit-sharing ratio, and accordingly the partnership agreement may state that employer's contributions should be prior charged to each relevant partner, and employees' contributions should be charged on an individual basis to the partners' current accounts.

If the above issues are dealt with properly, the chances of dispute are greatly reduced. This does not mean that other clauses, such as obligations, retirement, expulsion and restrictions, are not as important – indeed they are. However, if the partnership is conducted in the right spirit, the agreement should not take too long to draft and the practice should end up with a workable document.

As intimated earlier in this chapter it is now becoming more common for partnerships to include health professionals other than medical practitioners.

For the first time, non-clinicians have the opportunity to contract with the PCO in the capacity of a partner, and this will be recognised legally under the new contract. For those GPs who are reluctant to enter into a full partnership, as an alternative they may consider the salaried partnership option, which provides the necessary prestige but protects employment rights with none of the risks or responsibilities associated with unlimited liability partnership. Thus, the salaried partnership contract will state the master-servant relationship, hours of work, the paid leave for holidays, sickness arrangements, maternity and paternity rights, place of work, and the inability to hire and fire staff at will. In this way, a salaried partner would not be able to sign the PCO contract as such, but could appear on the practice letterhead with an appropriate indemnity from the equity partners.

Should a health professional, say a practice manager, become an equity partner, this will have a significant effect on the partnership deed. The following issues would need to be considered.

- Decision making – clinical decisions should be the responsibility of the clinicians only. So far as concerns non-clinicians, the agreement should be specific about relationships with clinicians.
- Voting rights given to non-clinicians should be restricted to non-clinical issues.
- Clinical partners may give non-clinical partners an indemnity in respect of third-party claims.
- Practice managers' responsibilities should be limited to areas such as finance, human resources, premises, etc.
- To whom employed medical staff account.
- The calculation of profit share.
- Time off, including that relating to professional development.
- Obligations and expulsions, i.e. corresponding commitments for other partners, for example professional obligations of nurses.
- Insurance – GPs must consider taking out comprehensive practice insurance, as well as individual clinical cover, to protect themselves, the practice as a whole and any non-clinical partners.
- The inclusion of the non-clinical partners in the NHS Pension Scheme.

For further guidance the reader is referred to the article in Chapter 16 entitled 'Partnerships – the legal status'.

CHAPTER 4

Practice accounts

Accurate accounts can be presented in a number of different ways. Poor presentation does not necessarily mean that the accounts are wrong. Indeed, there is no right or wrong way to present accounts, but accountants should strive to achieve best practice by presenting accounts that can be understood, contain all the information necessary to enable the partners to effectively run the finances of the practice, and to enable each and every partner to understand where they stand financially in relation to the practice.

The Association of Independent Specialist Medical Accountants (AISMA) regularly draws up a 'model' set of accounts, known as Upside Medical Practice, which purports to represent best practice at the time. These accounts are reproduced below. While 'Upside' has a 31 March year-end accounting date, practices can choose whatever accounting date they wish, but will need to take heed of the tax and superannuation effects of so doing. The 'overlapping' with the fiscal year is discussed further in Chapter 13.

So what are annual accounts used for and why are they so necessary? Here are some compelling reasons for drawing up meaningful annual accounts:

- to create an essential management tool by gauging the performance of the practice in order to maximise earnings
- to enable the practice to benchmark its performance against national and regional profiles in order to take corrective action and maximise income
- to provide a basis for calculating the partners' drawings and formulating future budgets
- to identify areas for achieving cost economies
- to comply with the partnership agreement
- to determine each partner's share of the partnership net assets and thereby maintain equity between them. Note that the net assets of the practice represent a mirror image of the partners' current accounts
- to attract new partners by providing them with information that will enable them to estimate their likely future earnings

- to enable the practice to calculate the amount due to an outgoing partner either on retirement or on leaving the practice for any other reason
- to support an application for new finance by providing financial institutions with sufficient information on which to base a decision. Note that this applies equally to individual partners as well as to the practice itself
- to provide a basis for calculating the tax liabilities of each partner and subsequently each of their superannuation contributions.

Given the above reasons for having annual accounts, the presentation of these accounts must be such as to achieve all the above objectives. Upside Medical Practice is, of course, a fictitious practice which can be used as a model for both PMS and GMS practices in the UK. The accounts are presented as follows.

UPSIDE MEDICAL PRACTICE
FINANCIAL STATEMENTS
FOR THE YEAR ENDED 31 MARCH 2008

CONTENTS   Page

PARTNERS
Dr A. Prodit
Dr I. Pokit
Dr S. Treatit
Dr M. Curit
Dr A. Preventit

SURGERY
Upside Surgery
Upside Road
Upside
UP1 4AB

UPSIDE MEDICAL PRACTICE
APPROVAL OF THE FINANCIAL STATEMENTS FOR THE YEAR
ENDED 31 MARCH 2008

In accordance with the terms of engagement we approve the financial statements set out on pages 3 to 15. We acknowledge our responsibility for the financial statements, including the appropriateness of the accounting basis set out in Note 18 and for providing RMT with all the information and explanations necessary for their compilation.

. . . .

Dr A. Prodit

. . . .

Dr I. Pokit

. . . .

Dr S. Treatit

. . . .

Dr M. Curit

. . . .

Dr A. Preventit

Approved on: 25 July 2008

UPSIDE MEDICAL PRACTICE
ACCOUNTANTS' REPORT ON THE UNAUDITED FINANCIAL
STATEMENTS FOR THE YEAR ENDED 31 MARCH 2008

In accordance with our terms of engagement we have compiled the financial statements of Upside Medical Practice set out on pages 3 to 15 from the accounting records and information and explanations provided to us.

The unaudited financial statements have been compiled on the accounting basis set out in note 18 to the financial statements. The financial statements are not intended to achieve full compliance with the provisions of UK Generally Accepted Accounting Practice.

This report is made to you in accordance with the terms of our engagement. Our work has been undertaken in order to prepare the financial statements that we have been engaged to compile, report to you that we have done so and state those matters that we have agreed to state to you in this report and for no other purpose. To the fullest extent permitted by law, we do not accept or assume any responsibility to anyone other than the partners of Upside Medical Practice, for our work, or for this report.

We have carried out this engagement in accordance with the technical guidance issued by the Institute of Chartered Accountants in England and Wales and have complied with the ethical guidance laid down by the Institute.

You have approved the financial statements for the year ended 31 March 2008 and have acknowledged your responsibility for them, for the appropriateness of the accounting basis and for providing all information and explanations necessary for their compilation.

We have not verified the accuracy or completeness of the accounting records or information and explanations you have provided to us and we do not, therefore, express any opinion on the financial statements.

RMT Accountants & Business Advisors
Gosforth Park Avenue
Newcastle upon Tyne
NE12 8EG

Approved on: 25 July 2008

UPSIDE MEDICAL PRACTICE
BALANCE SHEET AT 31 MARCH 2008

	Note	2008		2007	
		£	£	£	£
PARTNERS' FUNDS					
Property capital accounts	13		**115,000**		100,000
Partners' current accounts	14		**46,007**		47,974
			161,007		147,974
EMPLOYMENT OF FUNDS					
Tangible fixed assets	15		**262,625**		263,087
Loans	16		**(145,000)**		(160,000)
			117,625		103,087
CURRENT ASSETS					
Stock of drugs		**5,543**		5,279	
Debtors and prepayments		**117,415**		109,804	
Cash at bank and in hand		**67,926**		92,412	
		190,884		207,495	
LESS: CURRENT LIABILITIES					
Creditors and accrued charges		**42,117**		40,973	
Provision for income tax	17	**105,385**		121,635	
		147,502		162,608	
NET CURRENT ASSETS			**43,382**		44,887
			161,007		147,974

UPSIDE MEDICAL PRACTICE
DISTRIBUTION OF NET INCOME FOR THE YEAR ENDED
31 MARCH 2008

	Note	2008	2007
		£	£
PRACTICE INCOME (page 5)		630,092	648,742
PRIVATE INCOME	11	31,885	27,601
PERSONAL EXPENSES	12	(17,337)	(16,940)
PARTNERS' NET MEDICAL INCOME		644,640	659,403

Allocated as follows:

	Dr A. Prodit	Dr I. Pokit	Dr S. Treatit	Dr M. Curit	Dr A. Preventit	Total
	£	£	£	£	£	£
Seniority	11,457	6,989	6,785	6,785	3,504	35,520
Private income	400	7,600	7,125	6,650	10,110	31,885
Personal expenses	(3,526)	(3,286)	(3,319)	(3,590)	(3,616)	(17,337)
Notional rent	6,250	6,250	6,250	6,250	–	25,000
Property loan interest	(2,570)	(2,570)	(2,570)	(2,570)	–	(10,280)
Employer's superannuation on salaried post	(963)	241	241	241	240	–
Employer's superannuation	(16,135)	(17,405)	(16,912)	(16,878)	(16,808)	(84,138)
Balance distributed as follows	(5,087)	(2,181)	(2,400)	(3,112)	(6,570)	(19,350)
	132,798	132,798	132,798	132,798	132,798	663,990
To partners' current accounts (Note 14):	**127,711**	**130,617**	**130,398**	**129,686**	**129,228**	644,640
2007 EQUIVALENT	**132,210**	**135,120**	**130,488**	**131,371**	**130,214**	659,403

The profit-sharing ratios applied during the year were as follows:

	Dr A. Prodit	Dr I. Pokit	Dr S. Treatit	Dr M. Curit	Dr A. Preventit
01.04.07 to 31.03.08	20	20	20	20	20

UPSIDE MEDICAL PRACTICE
PRACTICE INCOME AND EXPENDITURE ACCOUNT FOR THE
YEAR ENDED 31 MARCH 2008

	Note	2008 £	2008 £	2007 £	2007 £
INCOME					
NHS income – GMS	1		1,102,240		1,074,352
Other NHS income	2		40,825		27,272
Employer's superannuation			(84,138)		(84,856)
Total NHS Income			1,058,927		1,016,768
Non-NHS income	3		35,195		32,312
Gross practice income			1,094,122		1,049,080
Reimbursement of expenses	4		59,081		66,196
Total Income			1,153,203		1,115,276
EXPENDITURE					
Staff costs	5	331,552		330,782	
Medical expenses	6	120,195		72,948	
Premises	7	35,163		28,564	
Administration	8	24,813		22,505	
Finance	9	10,741		10,897	
Depreciation	10	1,962		2,563	
			524,426		468,259
			628,777		647,017
Bank interest received			1,315		1,725
Net Practice Income (Page 4)			630,092		648,742

– 5 –

UPSIDE MEDICAL PRACTICE
NOTES TO THE FINANCIAL STATEMENTS AT 31 MARCH 2008

1 NHS income – GMS

	2008		2007
	£		£
General Medical Services			
GMS – global sum	536,828		531,580
Correction factor	147,401		147,401
Out of hours opt out	(32,210)		(31,895)
		652,019	647,086
PCO-administered income			
Locum cover	–		600
Seniority	35,520		31,372
		35,520	31,972
Enhanced services			
National			
Anticoagulation monitoring	6,443		6,912
IUCD fitting	907		876
Near patient testing	2,749		2,714
Directed			
Improved access scheme	21,908		10,637
Childhood immunisations – 2 year olds	17,004		16,974
Childhood immunisations – 5 year olds	5,311		5,252
Vaccinations – influenza, etc.	9,624		9,418
Minor surgery	7,112		6,393
Practice-based commissioning	15,953		11,136
Choice and booking	8,762		9,228
Local			
Nursing home cover	2,775		2,735
Smoking cessation	2,114		1,240
		100,662	83,515
Quality and outcome framework			
Aspiration and achievement	224,940		224,715
		224,940	224,715
Premises			
Notional rent	25,000		25,000
Rates, water and refuse	12,230		11,874
		37,230	36,874
Information management & technology			
Maintenance	275		–
		275	–
Dispensing and personal administration			
Dispensing fees	8,771		8,510
Drug costs	42,823		41,680
		51,594	50,190
		1,102,240	1,074,352

UPSIDE MEDICAL PRACTICE
NOTES TO THE FINANCIAL STATEMENTS AT 31 MARCH 2008
(continued)

2 Other NHS income

	2008	2007
	£	£
Dr Prodit – Training grant	7,325	7,024
Dr Prodit – Upside NHS Trust	8,600	8,534
Dr Curit – Clinical governance	16,000	5,750
Dr Preventit – Appraisals	8,900	5,964
	40,825	27,272

3 Other Non-NHS income

	2008	2007
	£	£
Insurance examinations, medicals and reports	28,521	25,914
Upside engineering	4,820	4,680
Cremation fees	1,354	1,468
Donations received	500	250
	35,195	32,312

4 Reimbursement of expenses

	2008	2007
	£	£
Registrar's salary and expenses	56,324	64,982
Staff training	400	–
Prescribing incentive savings – repairs	2,357	1,214
	59,081	66,196

5 Staff costs

	2008	2007
	£	£
Practice staff	242,011	232,703
Staff pension	31,731	30,511
Staff training	1,412	946
Staff uniforms	74	1,640
Registrar's salary and expenses	56,324	64,982
	331,552	330,782

UPSIDE MEDICAL PRACTICE
NOTES TO THE FINANCIAL STATEMENTS AT 31 MARCH 2008
(continued)

6 Medical expenses

	2008	2007
	£	£
Sundry medical supplies	4,928	4,811
Medical committee levy	2,763	2,432
Out of hours	252	244
Subscriptions including medical protection	23,244	22,350
Locum cover	1,100	2,900
Drugs	40,364	40,211
Salaried GP	47,544	–
	120,195	72,948

7 Premises

	2008	2007
	£	£
Rates, water and refuse	12,230	11,874
Heat and light	4,915	4,270
Insurance	2,617	2,515
Maintenance and repairs	7,844	2,709
Cleaning and laundry	7,557	7,196
	35,163	28,564

8 Administration

	2008	2007
	£	£
Telephone	5,230	4,984
Postage, stationery and technical literature	4,833	4,712
Equipment repairs	813	670
Computer expenses	784	644
Accountancy	7,050	6,756
Sundry expenses	3,008	2,993
Advertising	1,406	417
Legal and professional	429	118
Insurance	1,260	1,211
	24,813	22,505

9 Finance

	2008	2007
	£	£
Bank charges	461	433
Property loan interest	10,280	10,464
	10,741	10,897

UPSIDE MEDICAL PRACTICE
NOTES TO THE FINANCIAL STATEMENTS AT 31 MARCH 2008
(continued)

10 Depreciation

	2008	2007
	£	£
On fixtures, fittings and equipment	1,087	1,627
On computer equipment	875	936
	1,962	2,563

11 Partners' private income

	Dr A. Prodit	Dr I. Pokit	Dr S. Treatit	Dr M. Curit	Dr A. Preventit	Total
	£	£	£	£	£	£
Out of hours	–	4,750	–	–	9,100	13,850
Meeting fees	400	350	–	400	–	1,150
Medico-legal fees	–	–	7,125	6,250	–	13,375
Medical and research fees	–	2,500	–	–	1,010	3,510
	400	7,600	7,125	6,650	10,110	31,885

12 Partners' personal expenses

	Dr A. Prodit	Dr I. Pokit	Dr S. Treatit	Dr M. Curit	Dr A. Preventit	Total
	£	£	£	£	£	£
Spouses' salaries	–	–	600	750	–	1,350
Subscriptions	290	707	290	290	670	2,247
Courses and conferences	–	270	215	170	645	1,300
Sundry medical equipment	–	75	120	–	190	385
Locum insurance	1,759	484	361	376	299	3,279
Use of home	416	416	416	416	416	2,080
Motor expenses	633	807	788	1,014	963	4,205
Telephone	254	343	317	341	279	1,534
Stationery and computer expenses	174	184	212	233	154	957
	3,526	3,286	3,319	3,590	3,616	17,337

UPSIDE MEDICAL PRACTICE
NOTES TO THE FINANCIAL STATEMENTS AT 31 MARCH 2008
(continued)

13 Property capital accounts

	Dr A. Prodit	Dr I. Pokit	Dr S. Treatit	Dr M. Curit	Dr A. Preventit	Total
	£	£	£	£	£	£
At 1 April 2007	25,000	25,000	25,000	25,000	–	100,000
Transfer from partners' current accounts (Note 14)	3,750	3,750	3,750	3,750	–	15,000
At 31 March 2008	28,750	28,750	28,750	28,750	–	115,000

Represented by:
Freehold property (Note 15)   260,000
Less: loans (Note 16)   (145,000)
    115,000

14 Partners' current accounts

	Dr A. Prodit	Dr I. Pokit	Dr S. Treatit	Dr M. Curit	Dr A. Preventit	Total
	£	£	£	£	£	£
At 1 April 2007	9,258	9,478	9,831	9,650	9,757	47,974
Net income for the year (Page 4)	127,711	130,617	130,398	129,686	126,228	644,640
	136,969	140,095	140,229	139,336	135,985	692,614
Monthly drawings	60,000	58,800	59,700	59,700	61,400	299,600
Equalisation	5,258	5,478	5,831	5,650	5,757	27,974
Seniority drawn	11,457	6,989	6,785	6,785	3,504	35,520
Class 2 NIC	114	114	114	114	114	570
Superannuation						
– Standard paid	6,900	6,900	6,900	6,900	6,900	34,500
– Standard provided	15	559	348	334	303	1,559
– On other NHS income	516	–	–	–	–	516
Taxation – paid 2007/08	22,410	22,980	21,980	22,175	21,890	111,435
Taxation – provided 2007/08	20,570	21,140	21,940	21,485	20,250	105,385
Private income	400	7,600	7,125	6,650	10,110	31,885
Personal expenses	(3,526)	(3,286)	(3,319)	(3,590)	(3,616)	(17,337)
Transfer to property capital accounts (Note 13)	3,750	3,750	3,750	3,750	–	15,000
	127,864	131,024	131,154	129,953	126,612	646,607
At 31 March 2008	9,105	9,071	9,075	9,383	9,373	46,007

UPSIDE MEDICAL PRACTICE
NOTES TO THE FINANCIAL STATEMENTS AT 31 MARCH 2008
(continued)

15 Fixed assets

	Freehold property	Computer equipment	Fixtures, fittings and equipment	Total
	£	£	£	£
Cost				
At 1 April 2007	260,000	31,686	29,410	321,096
Additions	–	1,500	3,643	5,143
Reimbursements – prescribing incentive savings	–	–	(3,643)	(3,643)
At 31 March 2008	260,000	33,186	29,410	322,596
Depreciation				
At 1 April 2007	–	31,186	26,823	58,009
Charge for the year	–	875	1,087	1,962
At 31 March 2008	–	32,061	27,910	59,971
Net book value				
At 31 March 2008	**260,000**	**1,125**	**1,500**	**262,625**
At 31 March 2007	260,000	500	2,587	263,087

16 Loans

	Total
	£
At 1 April 2007	160,000
Interest charged for the year	10,280
	170,280
Repaid during the year	(25,280)
At 31 March 2008	145,000

The loan with Aisma Bank plc is secured on the freehold property. Interest is charged at 1% over base rate and is repayable in monthly instalments by 2016.

UPSIDE MEDICAL PRACTICE
NOTES TO THE FINANCIAL STATEMENTS AT 31 MARCH 2008
(continued)

17 Taxation

The financial statements for the year ended 31 March 2008 form the basis of the individual partners' liabilities to income tax on medical income for the year ended 5 April 2008, i.e. 2007/08. These liabilities have been provisionally calculated as follows:

	2007/08
Dr A. Prodit	42,980
Dr I. Pokit	44,120
Dr S. Treatit	43,920
Dr M. Curit	43,660
Dr A. Preventit	42,140
	£216,820

The above liabilities fall due for payment as follows:

	First payment on account 31/1/08	Second payment on account 31/7/08	Balance 31/1/09
Dr A. Prodit	22,410	22,410	(1,840)
Dr I. Pokit	22,980	22,980	(1,840)
Dr S. Treatit	21,980	21,980	(40)
Dr M. Curit	22,175	22,175	(690)
Dr A. Preventit	21,890	21,890	(1,640)
	£111,435	£111,435	£(6,050)

The overall liabilities of the individual partners for the year ended 5 April 2008 form the basis of their payments on account for the year ended 5 April 2009, i.e. 2008/09.

These payments on account, payable 31 January 2009 and 31 July 2009, are estimated as follows:

	Per Instalment
Dr A. Prodit	21,490
Dr I. Pokit	22,060
Dr S. Treatit	21,960
Dr M. Curit	21,830
Dr A. Preventit	21,070
	£108,410

UPSIDE MEDICAL PRACTICE
NOTES TO THE FINANCIAL STATEMENTS AT 31 MARCH 2008
(continued)

18 Principal accounting policies
Accounting convention
These financial statements have been prepared in accordance with the historical cost convention. The principal accounting policies which have been adopted within that convention are set out below.

Practice income
Practice income is the amount derived from the provision of medial services and the reimbursement of certain expenditure made by the local primary care organisations.

Depreciation
No depreciation is provided on the surgery premises.
For all other tangible assets, depreciation is calculated to write down their cost to their estimated residual values over the period of their estimated useful economic lives. The depreciation rates currently in use are:

Fixtures, fittings and equipment   – 15% straight line
Computer equipment   – 25% straight line

UPSIDE MEDICAL PRACTICE
NOTES TO THE FINANCIAL STATEMENTS AT 31 MARCH 2008
(continued)

19 Statistics

	National Profile	2008	2007
1 Average registered patient list	10,380	10,740	10,635
2 Average number of FTE GPs	5.00	5.00	5.00
3 Average patients per FTE GP	2,076	2,148	2,127
	£	£	£
4 Gross GMS/PMS income per patient			
Global sum/MPIG (after opt outs)	70.31	60.71	60.84
PCO-administered payments	3.45	3.31	3.01
Enhanced services	10.56	9.37	7.85
Quality and outcomes	21.16	20.94	21.13
Premises	8.17	3.47	3.47
Information management & technology	0.14	0.03	Nil
Dispensing	5.54	4.80	4.72
	119.33	102.63	101.02
5 Gross other NHS income per patient	5.16	5.20	4.06
6 Employer's superannuation per patient	(7.10)	(7.83)	(7.98)
7 Gross other non-NHS income per patient	5.81	4.85	4.14
8 Gross practice income per patient	123.20	104.85	101.24
9 Expenses per patient (after reimbursements)	67.08	44.82	39.24
10 Profit per patient	56.12	60.03	62.00
11 Quality and outcome points achievement	954	1,000	999
12 Gross GMS/PMS income per FTE GP:			
Global sum/MPIG (after opt outs)	145,960	130,404	129,417
PCO-administered payments	7,169	7,104	6,394
Enhanced services	21,923	20,132	16,703
Quality and outcomes	43,922	44,988	44,943
Premises	16,957	7,446	7,375
Information management & technology	290	55	–
Dispensing	11,508	10,319	10,038
	247,729	220,448	214,870

UPSIDE MEDICAL PRACTICE
NOTES TO THE FINANCIAL STATEMENTS AT 31 MARCH 2008
(continued)

19 Statistics (cont'd)

	National Profile	2008	2007
13 Gross practice income per FTE partner/(excluding reimbursements)			
– From GMS/PMS	247,729	220,448	214,870
– From other NHS sources	10,713	11,165	8,639
– From employer's superannuation	(14,730)	(16,828)	(16,971)
– From non-NHS sources	12,052	10,416	8,798
	255,764	225,201	215,336
14 Expenses per FTE partner			
– relating to NHS sources	132,702	91,821	80,046
– relating to non-NHS sources	6,562	4,453	3,410
	139,264	96,274	83,456
15 Profit per FTE partner			
– relating to NHS income	111,010	122,965	126,493
– relating to non-NHS income	5,490	5,963	5,388
	116,500	128,928	131,881
16 Expenses per patient (after reimbursement)			
Staff costs	32.90	25.50	25.01
Medical expenses	19.35	11.86	7.49
Premises	7.74	3.47	2.88
Administration	5.16	2.93	2.76
Financial	1.29	0.88	0.86
Depreciation	0.64	0.18	0.24
	67.08	44.82	39.24
	%	%	%
17 GMS/PMS income profile percentage			
Global sum/MPIG	58.90	59.15	60.23
PCO-administered payments	2.90	3.22	2.98
Enhanced services	8.80	9.13	7.77
Quality and outcomes	17.70	20.42	20.92
Premises	6.80	3.38	3.43
Information management & technology	0.10	0.02	Nil
Dispensing	4.80	4.68	4.67
	100.00	100.00	100.00
18 Percentage expenses to total income			
Staff costs	30.00	28.09	29.06
Medical expenses	15.00	10.75	6.97
Premises	6.00	3.14	2.68
Administration	4.00	2.66	2.56
Financial	1.00	0.80	0.80
Depreciation	0.50	0.17	0.22
	56.50	45.61	42.29

It is now worth considering the *raison d'être* of this layout. At the outset, comparative figures for the previous year are always shown in order to identify trends in income and expenditure. The first page, like any good book, merely lists the contents, the partners and the location of the surgeries. Pages 1 and 2 are the accountants' report and confirmation by the partners. The accounts belong to the partners who are responsible for their drafting. The accountants merely act as agents to prepare the accounts, but note that they are not engaged to conduct an audit.

Page 3 is the balance sheet of the practice, which is a snapshot of the practice net assets at midnight on the accounting date. The net assets are a mirror image of the property capital accounts and the partners' current accounts so that the latter reflects the partners' interest in the surgery premises and all of the other assets respectively. Subject to any revaluation of assets, the movement in the partners' current accounts year by year reflects the earnings of the partners, less what they draw during the year, so that in this example the earnings of the partners were just less than what they actually drew out. It is also worth referring to debtors and creditors, whereby the accounts recognise all income earned during the year, even if not yet received, and all expenditure incurred during the year, even if not yet paid. This is known as the 'accruals' concept, and GPs should therefore understand that the accounts are not just the receipts and payments during the year. It is extremely important that receipts and payments are allocated to the correct accounting period so that the objectives set out above are properly met. Finally, note that provision has been made for income tax, as it is the policy of this practice to meet the personal taxation liabilities of the partners. Legally, income tax is the responsibility of each individual partner and many practices choose to leave the payment to individual partners rather than take responsibility within the practice – both alternatives have merit and the choice is therefore left to each individual practice.

Page 4 discloses the partnership earnings and adjusts them for the private income and personal expenses of the individual partners to arrive at the partners' net medical income for the year. This is the 'cake', which is then divided up among the partners in accordance with the partnership agreement and variations thereto made from time to time. The transfer to partners' current accounts represents each partner's earnings before tax for the financial year. Some GPs and/or their accountants prefer not to disclose private income and personal expenses in the practice accounts at all, but to deal with them on a personal basis only. However, there are a number of compelling reasons for disclosing the private income and personal expenses of the partners, as follows.

- The 'benchmarking' against other practices and national and regional profiles can be damaged if like is not being compared with like. For example, one practice could treat subscriptions as a practice expense whereas another practice could treat subscriptions as a personal expense.
- Private income and personal expenses should be disclosed in the partnership tax return and not normally the individual partners' self-

assessment tax returns, unless it can be demonstrated that the activity in question is a separate trade.
- By comparing the expenses of each partner, items are unlikely to be omitted and claims understated.
- It saves preparing accounts for individual partners.
- It is in accordance with the concept of partnership, whereby partners are being open and honest with one another.
- It forms part of the superannuation calculations.

Page 5 is a summary of the partnership income and expenditure set out in standard format for easy comparison with other practices. Each item is referenced from note 1 to note 10 so that pages 6 to 9 inclusive provide the analysis of each of the items disclosed in page 5. Page 6 is, for example, the analysis of the GMS or PMS income set out under the headings appearing in the new contract. On page 7 non-GMS or PMS income is disclosed separately as NHS or non-NHS income, so that GPs are aware of which items are not considered to be superannuable (i.e. non-NHS income). Page 9 also analyses the partners' private income and personal expenses, the former of which has also to be split between NHS and non-NHS income for superannuation purposes.

Page 10 sets out the property capital accounts and the partners' current accounts in detail. The property capital accounts reflect the partners' equity in the surgery premises and it should be noted that Dr Preventit is not a property owner. The partners' current accounts reflect the partners' interest in all of the other net assets of the practice as set out in page 3. If earnings exceed drawings, their share in the net assets rises, but of course the converse is also true. The best way for a GP to understand their share of assets is to remember the following simple formula:

What I started the year with	A
Add: My earnings for the year (see page 4)	$+ \underline{B}$
	C
Less: What I have drawn during the year	$- D$
What I ended up with	$£ \underline{\underline{E}}$

The notes that support the balance sheet on page 3 are set out on page 11. Page 12 sets out the partners' tax position and is meant to give the partners as much warning as possible of future taxation liabilities. It also supports the provision made in the balance sheet on page 3. Page 13 is merely a statement of the accounting policies adopted.

Pages 14 and 15 convert the figures in the accounts to performance statistics and then compare the results not only to the previous year but also to the national profile benchmarking statistics prepared by AISMA. These two pages are extremely important in gauging the performance of the practice, as GPs will be able to identify where they have performed well and where they may need to direct some effort to improve performance. Obviously, in some instances corrective action cannot be taken as a shortfall may be due to a quirk of geography (e.g. dispensing and list sizes) or merely the ages of the partners (e.g. seniority). Nevertheless, the exercise should prove useful in any attempt to move a practice forward. The national profile statistics in Upside Medical Practice relate to non-dispensers in England.

The national profile statistics have been produced by AISMA using the survey into the accounts of AISMA GP clients for 2007, making adjustments for known changes, such as the Quality and Outcomes Framework, and using statistics provided by the Department of Health and equivalent body in Scotland. The national profile benchmarking statistics for 2007/08 were as follows for dispensing and non-dispensing practices:

Benchmarking Statistics 2007/08 – NON DISPENSERS

		England	Wales	Scotland	Northern Ireland	UK
1	Average registered patient list	6,487	6,250	5,284	4,986	6,299
2	Average number of FTE GPs (excluding salaried)	3.12	3.28	3.46	2.84	3.16
3	Average patients per FTE GP (excluding salaried GPs)	2,076	1,905	1,527	1,755	1,996
4	Gross GMS/PMS income per patient	£	£	£	£	£
	Global sum/MPIG (after opt outs)	70.31	65.23	67.75	61.07	67.02
	PCO-administered payments	3.45	3.31	4.41	4.09	3.46
	Enhanced services	10.56	9.82	11.29	11.62	10.24
	Quality and outcomes	21.16	21.23	24.96	24.04	20.94
	Premises	8.17	8.31	8.85	7.27	7.96
	Information management & technology	0.14	0.21	0.02	0.01	0.12
	Dispensing	5.54	5.67	0.02	–	4.54
		119.33	113.78	117.30	108.10	114.28
5	Gross other NHS income per patient	5.16	3.04	7.78	4.07	4.94
6	Employer's superannuation per patient	(7.10)	(6.69)	(7.78)	(7.56)	(6.79)
7	Gross other non-NHS income per patient	5.81	6.69	5.83	9.30	5.55

	England	Wales	Scotland	Northern Ireland	UK
8 Gross practice income per patient	123.20	116.82	123.13	113.91	117.98
9 Expenses per patient (after reimbursement)	(67.08)	(63.28)	(60.92)	(55.79)	(63.62)
10 Profit per patient	56.12	53.54	62.21	58.12	54.36
11 Quality and outcome points – achievement	968	965	982	975	969
12 Gross GMS/PMS income per FTE GP:	£	£	£	£	£
Global sum/MPIG (after opt outs)	145,960	124,271	103,457	107,174	133,763
PCO-administered payments	7,169	6,302	6,735	7,182	6,898
Enhanced services	21,923	18,715	17,244	20,392	20,443
Quality and outcomes	43,922	40,443	38,120	42,184	41,792
Premises	16,957	15,823	13,509	12,772	15,895
Information management & technology	290	409	32	16	243
Dispensing fees, on cost, and PA	11,508	10,787	18	–	9,061
	247,729	216,750	179,115	189,720	228,095
13 Gross practice income per FTE partner (excluding reimbursements)					
– from GMS/PMS	247,729	216,750	179,115	189,720	228,095
– from other NHS sources	10,713	5,795	11,875	7,140	9,864
– from employer's superannuation	(14,730)	(12,750)	(11,875)	(13,260)	(13,562)
– from non-NHS sources	12,052	12,750	8,906	16,320	11,097
	255,764	222,545	188,021	199,920	235,494
14 Expenses per FTE partner					
– relating to NHS income	132,702	113,639	88,615	89,927	121,010
– relating to non-NHS income	6,562	6,906	4,406	7,993	5,984
	139,264	120,545	93,021	97,920	126,994
15 Profit per FTE partner					
– relating to NHS income	110,010	96,156	90,500	93,673	103,387
– relating to non-NHS income	5,490	5,844	4,500	8,327	5,113
	116,500	102,000	95,000	102,000	108,500
16 Expenses per patient (after reimbursement)					
– Staff costs	32.90	31.64	32.40	30.22	31.50

	England	Wales	Scotland	Northern Ireland	UK
– Medical expenses	19.35	17.65	11.67	9.30	17.91
– Premises	7.74	6.08	9.07	5.81	7.41
– Administration	5.16	5.48	5.83	8.14	4.94
– Financial	1.29	1.82	1.30	1.74	1.24
– Depreciation	0.64	0.61	0.65	0.58	0.62
	67.08	63.28	60.92	55.79	63.62
17 GMS/PMS income profile percentage	%	%	%	%	%
Global sum/MPIG	58.9	57.3	57.8	56.5	58.6
PCO-administered payments	2.9	2.9	3.8	3.8	3.0
Enhanced services	8.8	8.6	9.6	10.7	9.0
Quality and outcomes	17.7	18.7	21.3	22.3	18.3
Premises	6.8	7.3	7.5	6.7	7.0
Information management & technology	0.1	0.2	–	–	0.1
Dispensing fees, on cost, and PA	4.8	5.0	–	–	4.0
	100.0	100.0	100.0	100.0	100.0
18 Percentage expenses to total income					
Staff costs	30.0	30.0	30.0	28.0	30.0
Medical expenses	15.0	14.5	9.0	8.0	14.5
Premises	6.0	5.0	7.0	5.0	6.0
Administration	4.0	4.5	4.5	7.0	4.0
Financial	1.0	1.5	1.0	1.5	1.0
Depreciation	0.5	0.5	0.5	0.5	0.5
	56.6	56.0	52.0	50.0	56.00

Benchmarking Statistics 2007/08 – DISPENSERS

	England	Wales	Scotland	Northern Ireland	UK
1 Average registered patient list	6.487	6,250	5,284	n/a	6,299
2 Average number of FTE GPs (excluding salaried)	3.12	3.28	3.46	n/a	3.16
3 Average patients per FTE GP (excluding salaried GPs)	2,076	1,905	1,527	n/a	1,996
4 Gross GMS/PMS income per patient	£	£	£	£	£
Global sum/MPIG (after opt outs)	64.99	62.01	71.11	n/a	66.12

	England	Wales	Scotland	Northern Ireland	UK
PCO-administered payments	3.34	3.43	6.29	n/a	3.47
Enhanced services	11.26	9.56	12.74	n/a	11.40
Quality and outcomes	19.55	19.11	21.50	n/a	19.92
Premises	8.31	8.40	14.88	n/a	8.62
Information management & technology	0.12	0.22	0.14	n/a	0.12
Dispensing	72.84	54.86	68.31	n/a	72.99
	180.41	157.59	194.97	n/a	182.64
5 Gross other NHS income per patient	3.72	4.98	14.83	n/a	4.73
6 Employer's superannuation per patient	(8.37)	(7.48)	(8.47)	n/a	(8.52)
7 Gross other non-NHS income per patient	5.58	5.81	5.30	n/a	5.69
8 Gross practice income per patient	181.34	160.90	206.63	n/a	184.54
9 Expenses per patient (after reimbursement)	(114.38)	(98.70)	(130.34)	n/a	(116.40)
10 Profit per patient	66.96	62.20	76.29	n/a	68.14
11 Quality and outcome points – achievement	975	966	978	n/a	975
12 Gross GMS/PMS income per FTE GP:					
Global sum/MPIG (after opt outs)	134,921	118,126	108,581	n/a	131,982
PCO-administered payments	6,926	6,536	9,602	n/a	6,929
Enhanced services	23,373	18,210	19,455	n/a	22,746
Quality and outcomes	40,591	36,399	32,827	n/a	39,765
Premises	17,254	16,006	22,716	n/a	17,207
Information management & technology	240	411	213	n/a	247
Dispensing fees, on cost, and PA	151,223	104,512	104,328	n/a	145,681
	374,528	300,200	297,722	n/a	364,557
13 Gross practice income per FTE partner (excluding reimbursements)					
– from GMS/PMS	374,528	300,200	297,722	n/a	364,557
– from other NHS sources	7,722	9,480	22,653	n/a	9,444
– from employer's superannuation	(17,375)	(14,220)	(12,944)	n/a	(17,000)

	England	Wales	Scotland	Northern Ireland	UK
– from non-NHS sources	11,583	11,060	8,090	n/a	11,333
	376,458	306,520	315,521	n/a	368,334
14 Expenses per FTE partner					
– relating to NHS sources	230,152	181,236	193,918	n/a	225,186
– relating to non-NHS sources	7,306	6,784	5,103	n/a	7,148
	237,458	188,020	199,021	n/a	232,334
15 Profit per FTE partner					
– relating to NHS income	134,723	114,224	113,513	n/a	131,815
– relating to non-NHS income	4,277	4,276	2,987	n/a	4,185
	139,000	118,500	116,500	n/a	136,000
16 Expenses per patient (after reimbursement)					
– Staff costs	41.85	36.50	47.69	n/a	42.59
– Medical expenses	55.80	46.44	59.34	n/a	57.73
– Premises	7.44	5.81	13.77	n/a	7.57
– Administration	6.51	5.80	6.36	n/a	5.68
– Financial	1.86	3.32	2.12	n/a	1.89
– Depreciation	0.92	0.83	1.06	n/a	0.94
	114.38	98.70	130.34	n/a	116.40
17 GMS/PMS income profile percentage	%	%	%	%	%
Global sum/MPIG	36.0	39.3	36.5	n/a	36.2
PCO-administered payments	1.8	2.2	3.2	n/a	1.9
Enhanced services	6.2	6.1	6.5	n/a	6.2
Quality and outcomes	10.8	12.1	11.0	n/a	10.9
Premises	4.6	5.3	7.6	n/a	4.7
Information management & technology	0.1	0.1	0.1	n/a	0.1
Dispensing fees, on cost, and PA	40.5	34.9	35.1	n/a	40.0
	100.0	100.0	100.0	n/a	100.0
18 Percentage expenses to total income					
Staff costs	25.0	25.0	25.0	n/a	25.0
Medical expenses	30.0	28.0	28.0	n/a	30.5
Premises	4.0	3.5	6.5	n/a	4.0
Administration	3.5	3.5	3.0	n/a	3.0
Financial	1.0	2.0	1.0	n/a	1.0
Depreciation	0.5	0.5	0.5	n/a	0.5
	64.0	62.5	64.0	n/a	64.0

The practice accounts are therefore quite complex and extremely detailed. It is not surprising that many GPs and practice managers are often confused as to what information their accountant will need in order to prepare accounts such as those of Upside Medical Practice. To assist practices with this task, here is a suggested checklist of records that you should supply to your accountants annually.

Tick box
when complete

1 (a) Cashbook, all receipts and payments fully written up and analysed for the whole financial year, all columns totalled and cross-additions checked with cheque and cash payments clearly identified. Bank reconciliations if applicable. ☐
   or
   (b) Computerised print-out of receipts and payments together with audit trail for full year and transaction history supported by CD of files. ☐

2 Bank statements for all bank accounts and/or building society accounts covering the financial year and the month after the accounting date. ☐

3 Cheque book stubs and pay-in slips for the entire accounting year. ☐

4 The personal expenses/private income checklist for every partner for the financial year. ☐

5 A list of amounts you owe (creditors). ☐

6 All purchase invoices relating to the financial year and to creditors (5 above), together with suppliers' statements if applicable. ☐

7 Copies of any new finance/HP agreements. ☐

8 Details of any loans and a copy of the agreement. ☐

9 All vouchers relating to the financial year in support of non-GMS income received. ☐

10 Payslips in respect of any hospital or other outside appointments earned by the practice in the financial year. ☐

11 All health authority vouchers relating to the financial year and for the quarter thereafter in support of GMS income and reimbursements received or PMS income. ☐

12 A list of amounts owed to you (debtors). ☐

13 Your stock of drugs at the year-end accounting date. ☐

14 Your petty cash record for the financial year together with all vouchers, and a note of cash and cheques held but not banked at the year-end accounting date. ☐

15 A payroll summary for the financial year together with a copy of last completed form P35. ☐

16 Copies of relevant correspondence from the health authority
   in support of items paid direct by the health authority on
   behalf of the practice, such as rent, rates, water, etc.   ❐
17 All PCT vouchers relating to the financial year in support of
   cash-limited reimbursements received.   ❐
18 A list of items purchased out of 'savings' derived from
   fundholding, prescribing incentives, etc. for the financial year.   ❐

The same information should be supplied irrespective of whether the practice
is GMS or PMS.

   If the above information is to be supplied to the practice accountant,
practices must maintain accounting records which enable them to produce this
information with the minimum of effort. The majority of practices now choose
to operate a computerised accounting system and there is a great deal of software
available on the market. However, the key to success is to ensure that the software
can perform all the functions of a manual accounting system. Thus, the most
commonly required functions are:
• receipts and payments analysis
• NHS analysis
• ability to cope with a number of bank, building society, loan and petty
  cash accounts
• facilities for inter-account transfers
• direct debit or standing order facilities
• ability to cope with any accounting period
• bank reconciliation facilities
• print-outs of data available
• back-up capabilities.

Whether the records are manual or computerised, the analysis headings should
broadly follow the accounts headings set out in the Upside Medical Practice
earlier. Thus, the following records are recommended.
1 Bank receipts
   – total amount of receipt
   – PCT income
   – dispensing income
   – net remuneration from outside appointments
   – private patient fees
   – sundry fees such as medicals, reports, police fees, cremation
     fees, etc.
   – other income such as rent received, donations, sale of equipment, etc.
   – amount banked.
2 Bank payments
   – total amount of cheque, direct debit or standing order

- salaries, PAYE, and NIC and pensions for staff, registrars, retainers, salaried GPs, career start and assistants
- locum cover and deputising costs
- subscriptions
- surgery medical supplies (consumables)
- drugs for prescribing
- rent, rates, water and refuse
- heating and lighting
- insurance
- maintenance and repairs
- telephone and fax
- equipment hire and maintenance
- printing, postage, stationery and technical literature
- laundry and cleaning
- professional fees
- advertising
- general expenses
- cheques for petty cash
- bank interest and charges
- loan repayments, leasing costs and hire purchase payments
- computer expenses
- capital expenditure (computers, equipment, furniture, etc.)
- partners' drawings, including tax and NIC.

3 PCT record
- GMS/PMS lump sum
- PCO-administered income such as GP retainer, locum cover, seniority, etc.
- national enhanced services
- directed enhanced services
- local enhanced services
- Quality and Outcomes Framework
- premises (rent, rates, refuse, clinical waste, etc.)
- information management and technology (computer maintenance, etc.)
- dispensing (dispensing fees and on-cost, reimbursements).

4 Dispensing record
- date received
- monthly prescriptions dispensed
- basic price
- dispensing fees
- VAT (on personally administered drugs)
- prescription charges collected
- adjustments
- discount
- total due

- advance received
- deduction for advance recovered
- total received
- number of forms
- number of prescriptions
- number disallowed.

5 Outside appointments record
  - name of doctor and hospital or employer
  - month salary received
  - gross salary
  - PAYE and NIC
  - superannuation
  - other deductions
  - net salary received (per bank receipts book).

6 Petty cash record
  - total receipt
  - cash from main bank account
  - other income
  - total payment
  - various analysis columns to suit.

7 Bank statement file.

8 Income voucher file.

9 PCT schedules (both GMS and PMS) (including QMAS reports).

10 Expenditure voucher file.

11 Salaries records
  - gross salary
  - deductions for PAYE, pension contributions, Class 1 NIC
  - net salary
  - SSP/SMP if applicable
  - Class 1 NIC (employer's share)
  - employer's pension contributions.

12 Appointments record
  - insurance medicals (name of patient, date, fee and date paid)
  - private fees
  - other fees.

The above records should be sufficient even to cope with dispensing practices. However, the annual accounts of dispensing practices should disclose an additional note that separates out the dispensing activities from the other activities of the practice so that GPs can identify properly where their earnings are coming from. The additional note might be set out as follows.

Dispensary

The practice operates a dispensary, the results of which are included in these financial statements as follows:

	2008	2007
	£	£
Dispensing fees	82,820	80,800
Drug reimbursements	289,467	282,406
Total drug income	372,287	363,206
Drugs purchased	(214,920)	(207,652)
Dispensing profit	157,367	155,554
The total drug income above comprises the following:		
Basic price	317,579	309,833
Dispensing fees	82,820	80,800
VAT	8,228	8,027
Discount	(36,340)	(35,454)
	372,287	363,206

To ensure that the records are effective and accurate, practices need to set up effective financial management systems which should be documented and adhered to. A fully systemised practice is a much safer business than one relying totally on what is in the practice manager's head. To assist practices setting up a financial management system, a suggested financial system checklist is shown in the box below.

Collecting fees
- How are fees collected for relevant services?
- Does the system ensure the following:
  - every person who should be charged is charged?
  - those who are charged actually pay?
  - income (whether in the form of cash or cheque) is banked regularly?
  - someone who is not involved in the receipt or banking of the funds reconciles the expected receipts with the actual receipts and confirms that they are correctly banked?

Petty cash
- Does the system ensure the following:
  - payments can only be made with approved petty cash slips?
  - no one can reimburse themselves out of the petty cash without someone else checking it?
  - the total of cash and receipts in the tin always matches the agreed

petty cash level (whether this is checked daily, weekly or monthly will depend on the level of petty cash expenditure)?
— no cash fees can find their way into petty cash (or just be used for paying expenses)?
— the key to the petty cash tin is kept in a safe place?

Cheque payments

- Are cheques drawn only by an authorised person and the cheque books kept securely?
- Is it clear who can sign for what? Normally, one partner's signature will be required for amounts up to, say, £500, and two for larger amounts. The practice manager should not normally be permitted to be sole signatory.
- When cheques are signed, are they accompanied by authorised invoices?
- Are all invoices authorised by an appropriate person?
- Is the cheque number written on the invoice (to prevent double payment)?
- If payments are by Internet rather than by cheque are similar controls in place?

Payroll

- Is the payroll prepared in-house or outsourced?
- Does someone not involved in payroll check the names from time to time?
- What system is there to check that the correct pay rates are being used?
- Is there a system to check hours claimed for?
- Do overtime hours have to be properly authorised?

Income

- Is there a system to check that all income due is actually received by the practice?
- How does the practice manager know what is to be expected? Is communication with the doctors adequate?

Actual income and expenditure compared to budget

- Are management accounts produced and compared to the practice budget?
- Are major variances investigated?
- Is this reviewed on an ongoing basis or only when the accounts are prepared after the year end?

Staff appointment and training to avoid financial risk

- Are references always taken up?
- Does induction training emphasise the use of systems, and does the inductee have access to the systems manual?
- Do regular appraisals look at systems and efficiencies and continually update the systems?

Medical practice accounting has certainly become more complex in recent years. It is no wonder that many accountants have had to specialise in medical practice finance, and GPs are recommended to use a specialist if at all possible. At the end of the day, it is 'horses for courses' – the writer would not accept instructions from a farmer!

CHAPTER 5

The contract for services

There is an enormous amount of documentation relating to GPs' pay under the new contract and to explain it fully in prose could fill a book on its own. In an attempt to highlight the key points only, this chapter has been written in 'bullet point' format deliberately to enable the reader to grasp the essence of income sources and then refer to the voluminous and various guidelines only when appropriate.

OVERVIEW OF CONTRACT INCOME SOURCES

- Implementation of the new contract is effective from 1 April 2004.
- Values of services will mostly be nationally determined, with the exception of local enhanced services (LES).
- Payments are practice not practitioner based; they are paid by a primary care organisation to a contractor.
- The new general medical services contract payments are outlined in the Statement of Financial Entitlements, for 2005/06 as published on 30 March 2005 and updated on 8 June 2005.
- The 2006/07 contract negotiations were confirmed on 20 December 2005 with no uplift to any element of the contract for inflation or cost pressures.
- The latest consolidated version of the SFE was published on 1 December 2007.
- The SFE may be revised at any time and may have a retrospective effect.
- The Department of Health is responsible for the information contained therein.
- Amendments to the SFE are published periodically along with effective implementation dates.
- The content of the standard GMS contract has been agreed between the DoH, General Practitioners Committee (GPC) and NHS Confederation and was amended with effect from 28 January 2008. It is applicable to all

new contracts issued after that date. Existing contracts have to be updated to effect the variations.

THE GLOBAL SUM (GS)

- This covers the expenses and profits related to the delivery of essential and additional services, including staff costs. It is an annual sum, adjusted quarterly and paid monthly.
- Payments are conditional on the contractor making required information available to the PCO.
- It represents between 50% and 66% of a practice's total income, excluding premises funding, in 2004/05.
- This percentage falls in 2005/06 as funding from enhanced services and the Quality and Outcomes Framework (QOF) increases.
- GS depends on list size, relative workload and costs of delivery as determined by the Carr-Hill formula. An adjustment is made to take account of the registered population compared to the weighted population.
- As this is not a static situation, the Technical Steering Committee have been charged with carrying out annual workload surveys and collation of expenses data, which will be used to price the contract from April 2006.
- It is updated every quarter for list size and list profile changes.
- Minimum practice income guarantee (MPIG) applies to ensure practices receive as much for essential and additional services in 2004/05 and beyond as they did in 2003/04, i.e. their global sum equivalent (GSE).
- The mapping of the GSE is given in Annex D of the Statement of Financial Entitlements (SFE).
- The difference between the GSE and the global sum (GS) is the correction factor (CF).
- The GS or MPIG covers 21 different old Red Book equivalent payments, including amounts previously dealt with as a direct reimbursement.
- The GS is adjusted for any opt outs.

CALCULATION OF ADJUSTED GLOBAL SUM MONTHLY PAYMENTS (GSMP)

- If, where an initial GSMP for the financial year has been calculated, the relevant GMS contract stipulates that the contractor is not to provide one or more of the additional or out-of-hours services listed in column 1 of the table below, the PCO is to calculate an adjusted GSMP for that contractor as follows.
- If the contractor is not going to provide:
  (a) one of the additional or out-of-hours services listed in column 1 of the table, the contractor's adjusted GSMP will be its initial GSMP reduced

by the percentage listed opposite the service it is not going to provide in column 2 of the table;

(b) more than one of the additional or out-of-hours services listed in column 1 of the table, an amount is to be deducted in respect of each service it is not going to provide. The value of the deduction for each service is to be calculated by reducing the contractor's initial GSMP by the percentage listed opposite that service in column 2 of the table, without any other deductions from the initial GSMP first being taken into account. The total of all the deductions in respect of each service is then deducted from the initial GSMP to produce the adjusted GSMP.

Additional or out-of-hours services	Percentage of initial GSMP
Cervical screening services	1.1
Child health surveillance	0.7
Minor surgery	0.6
Maternity medical services	2.1
Contraceptive services	2.4
Childhood immunisations and pre-school boosters	1.0
Vaccinations and immunisations	2.0
Out-of-hours services	6.0

- The GS payments are reduced by a deduction for the estimated costs of both the employer (14%) and the employee (6%) superannuation contributions together with added years if applicable.

ESSENTIAL SERVICES
- Responsive care for registered patients and temporary patients who are or who believe themselves to be ill from conditions where recovery is expected, terminally ill or suffering from chronic disease.
- Care to be delivered in the manner determined by the practice in discussion with the patient.
- Defined in the NHS (GMS Contracts) Regulations 2004, part 5, paragraph 15(3).

ADDITIONAL SERVICES
These include the following:
- child health surveillance
- contraceptive services
- cervical screening
- vaccinations and immunisations

- childhood immunisation and booster
- non-intra-partum maternity services
- curettage, cautery and cryotherapy minor surgery
- temporary or permanent opt out or subcontracting of these services is possible.

STAFF

The more important issues to note are the following.
- The contractor is now responsible for the entire cost of employment, including employer NI and pension contributions.
- The GS is calculated to include average amounts to cover these expenses.
- Staff management and utilisation will become very important to the way practice profits are generated in the future.
- Job descriptions may need review and revision.
- *Agenda for Change*, although not compulsory in general practice, and currently unfunded, is having a cost impact on many practices.

OUT OF HOURS

The main features are as follows.
- From 1 January 2005 responsibility for out of hours rests with the PCO.
- The out-of-hours period is 6.30 pm to 8.00 am Monday to Friday, all day Saturday, Sunday and Bank (Public) Holidays.
- Providers of out-of-hours services must meet the Carson Report quality standards.
- Practices may choose not to opt out of this responsibility and can subcontract to other providers.
- The opt-out cost is 6% of the GS.
- In exceptional areas of extreme rurality or remoteness practices may be unable to opt out. A support package should then be agreed with the PCO.
- Circumstances for in-hours visits have been clarified in the new contract.
- Some practices, due to workforce difficulties, may temporarily or permanently contract the PCO to provide in-hours visiting.
- Funds will transfer from the practice to cover this.
- Reviews of patient transport arrangements will be made.

SENIORITY

The system has been materially changed under the new contract and the new rules can be summarised as follows.
- Seniority payments depend on the number of years each individual GP has worked in the NHS, i.e. reckonable service.
- NHS superannuation records will be used to verify this, together

with evidence of GP locum work undertaken prior to it becoming superannuable.
- The chart of seniority payments is in Chapter 13 of the SFE.
- Seniority is paid in proportion to superannuable earnings by comparison with the national average. The national average will not be known until superannuation certificates are aggregated many months after the end of the financial year.
- If a GP's figure is more than two thirds of the national average then full seniority is paid.
- It is reduced to 60% of the maximum payment if earnings are between one-third and two-thirds.
- No payment is made if earnings are below one-third.
- For 2004/05 the payment will be based on the proportion received in 2003/04 unless the practice circumstances have changed.
- If a GP is disadvantaged by being in a low-earning practice, an appeal can be made to the PCO for an upward-only adjustment to the seniority pay.
- GPs are eligible for seniority if they have been in the post for two years.
- Retrospective over/underpayments can occur.
- As at September 2008, no final national averages have been published. Interim estimated figures are in use.

OTHER PCO FUNDING

This is available on a discretionary basis to cover locum payments, flexible careers scheme, retainer's scheme, returner scheme and prolonged study leave. Increases in the maximum reimbursements came into effect for 2006/07.

ENHANCED SERVICES
- Prices of directed and national enhanced services are set nationally.
- PCOs have a minimum guaranteed expenditure floor set nationally for these.
- LMCs have to approve that the services funded from this 'floor' meet the definition of enhanced services.
- PCOs have a legal obligation to commission and pay for directed enhanced services (DES).
- Volume of work, specification for the work, quality and monitoring and payment for work will all be agreed in advance and an appropriate contract signed between the PCO and the practice.
- Local development schemes, improving primary care incentive scheme, services previously delivered under HSG(96)31, GPs with Special Interests (GPwSIs) and schemes to improve patient access have been subsumed into enhanced services.

NATIONAL ENHANCED SERVICES (NES)

Optional services, with national specifications and benchmark prices, shift services from secondary to primary care. Initially, these were the following:

- anti-coagulation monitoring
- enhanced care of the homeless
- intra-partum care
- fitting of intra uterine devices (IUDs)
- minor injury services, in special geographic circumstances in-hours service at a fee of £1,032.25 retainer plus £51.61 per patient episode for 2004/05; the volume of claims may be capped
- specialised services for MS patients
- specialised sexual health services
- services to alcohol misusers
- services to drug misusers
- near-patient testing.
- immediate care and first response care; in special geographic circumstances this provides for practices to augment the ambulance service
- specialist care to patients with depression.

If the PCO does not contract with a practice to provide an NES the practice should give notice of its intention to withdraw from providing that service.

DIRECTED ENHANCED SERVICES

These are services to be commissioned by PCOs, with national specifications and benchmark prices, as follows.

- Care and treatment of patients who have a history of violence.
- Childhood vaccinations and immunisations for age two and under and pre-school boosters; practices have preferred provider status, payable quarterly in arrears.
- Flu immunisations, payment for each patient immunised, targets to aim for, separate payments for over 65s and at-risk under 65s.
- Minor surgery, paid as an item of service or as a block contract, £40 for injections, £80 for cutting surgery.
- Improved access, available only until 2005/06; practices have preferred provider status. There are different targets in each country. Payment per patient on the list is 50% at the start of the year, with the balance at end if achieved level of access.
- For 2006/07 50 QOF points previously available for access and their associated funding are amalgamated into the new access DES.
- There are different targets in each country. Payment per patient on the list is 50% at the start of the year, with the balance at end if achieved level of access.
- For 2006/07 a choice and booking DES rewards practices at 95p per

registered patient if patients have been offered choice (measured via an independent survey) and booking has been effected through the choose and book software. This cost will be reviewed in 2007/08.

- Practice-based commissioning (PBC) is a one-year DES introduced for 2006/07 and is a two part payment. The first part is 95p per registered patient to encourage involvement by drafting a plan. The second payment will be awarded at 95p per registered patient if the plan is delivered. This latter is paid as an alternative to, not in addition to, any saving made.
- A one-off DES for adopting information management and technology (IM&T) systems to implement the Connecting for Health programme was introduced for 2006/07. The total payable of £1.33 per patient is likely to be spread over two years.

LOCAL ENHANCED SERVICES

These are discretionary services determined by local negotiation between PCOs and providers.

THE QUALITY AND OUTCOMES FRAMEWORK (QOF)

Much has already been written on this subject but it is still worth summarising the major issues, as follows.

- Participation in the QOF is voluntary.
- Each quality point has a value of £77.50 in 2004/05 for an average practice with 5891 patients (in England) with average morbidity.
- Practice-level prevalence will be incorporated into the payments for each disease in the clinical domain in the achievement payment.
- The value increased to £124.60 in 2005/06 and currently remains at this level.
- Aspiration payments are paid in 12 equal monthly instalments; for 2008/09 these are equal to 70% of the previous year's achievement.
- The level of quality achieved will be assessed after 31 March and a balancing achievement payment made no later than 30 June.
- There are four domains: clinical, organisational, additional services and patient experience; 2006/07 introduced new clinical areas and tougher thresholds.
- Reward is given for breadth of achievement across the whole framework.
- Each domain contains a range of areas described by key indicators and each indicator is divided into structure, process and outcome.
- The framework will be updated for changes in the evidence base.
- There were 1000 points available plus an extra 50 points for achieving access targets in 2005/06. The 50 QOF points for access have since been removed from QOF and reallocated into DES income.
- If a practice does not achieve at least 150 points, an amount is withheld

from the practice's GS as follows: the PCO must withhold from the contractor the amount produced by multiplying

(a) 150; by

(b) the amount specified as the value of each achievement point in a calculation of an achievement payment for the financial year to which the achievement points total relates; by

(c) the contractor's Contractor Population Index that is, or would be, used for the calculation of any achievement payment due to the contractor in respect of that financial year (the contractor will, in any event, receive an achievement payment in respect of the points it does score for that financial year).

However, if the contractor's GMS contract either takes effect during, or is terminated before the end of, that financial year, the amount to be withheld pursuant to paragraph 2.16 is to be adjusted by the fraction produced by dividing the number of days during which the financial year for which its GMS contract had effect by 365.

- Exception reporting is taken into account.
- The framework effects a collection of data.
- The Quality Management Analysis System (QMAS) extracts and aggregates the disease register information from a practice's clinical system.
- PCOs will visit every practice annually to discuss performance.
- Use of good computer systems to manage and record information will be paramount.
- Use of preferred Read codes as per the NHS website www. connectingforhealth.nhs.uk/systemsandservices/data/readcodes or www. ceppc.org/guidelines in Scotland.
- Proposed changes to the QOF for 2008/09 have been published but the SFE has not yet been updated to reflect them. 58.5 points will be reallocated to reward patient satisfaction with access.
- National prevalence day will be set as 31 March from 2009.

PREMISES

Premises costs payable under GMS contracts are dealt with in the Primary Medical Services (Premises Costs) (England) Directions 2004. The following paragraph deals with the applications of these Directions.

APPLICATIONS

- Proposals for one-stop developments are more likely to receive funding approval than simpler existing surgery arrangements.
- PCOs are required to consider applications for financial assistance towards premises development and improvement for the delivery of primary

medical services, on receipt of architects' plans and competitive
tenders.
- Any such plans must be Disability Discrimination Act (DDA) 1995
  compliant, should have regard to the standards provided in Primary
  and Social Care Premises: planning and design guidance www.pcc.nhs.
  uk/planning-and-design-guidance.php and should have regard to the
  minimum standards for practice premises as laid out in Schedule 1 of the
  Directions.
- Practices should involve their LMC in discussions and seek professional
  specialist advice.
- Funds for development are held by a PCO lead within a strategic health
  authority.
- Minimum standards are set out for surgery premises.
- Third-party developers are frequently more involved through Private
  Finance Initiative (PFI) projects and lease arrangements.
- Suggested reading in this area: *The Future of GP Practice Premises: guidance for
  GPs* at www.bma.org.uk.
- Where PCOs committed prior to 1 April 2004 to provide financial
  assistance on or after 1 April 2005 towards (a) building new premises, (b)
  purchase of new premises, (c) development of new premises or (d) by way
  of improvement grants, those commitments must be met.

IMPROVEMENT GRANTS

- Improvement grants of 33–66% are available, subject to PCO discretion
  and budget constraints, for extensions and enlargements, improving access
  to comply with the DDA 1995, improving lighting, ventilation or heating,
  reasonable extension of telephone systems, provision of car parking,
  adaptations to meet the needs of children, the elderly or the infirm and
  improvements to fire precaution and security.
- Professional fees of surveyors/architects are now reimbursable, as are
  project-management costs.

NOTIONAL AND COST RENT

- Notional rent payments remain but, where the NHS has contributed
  capital to a building or refurbishment at any time after 18 September 2003,
  the notional rent is abated for 10 years on a proportional basis.
- Cost rent is renamed borrowing costs reimbursement.
- Both these payments form part of the guaranteed baseline funding of
  PCOs and will be uplifted each year for property cost inflation.
- The borrowing costs reimbursement is paid until the loan is repaid or
  notional rent exceeds it.
- Any changes to the borrowing arrangements must be notified to the PCO.

- It is possible to receive both cost and notional rent on premises where an extension has been constructed, or where a GP tenant has carried out improvements to a leasehold property.
- Reference should be made to the NHS (GMS-Premises Costs) Directions 2004.
- Branch surgeries open 20 hours per week and staffed to provide a full range of services will be eligible for premises reimbursement including the costs of a real-time land-line computer link.

FLEXIBILITIES

- Flexibilities have been introduced to assist with problems that can arise on disposal of existing premises, but various conditions must be satisfied.
- These include grants of 100% of negative equity; mortgage redemption fees; grants to cover loans for those in a situation where there is a move to approved leasehold premises.
- Grants may also be made to reconvert old surgery premises to residential use by a registered social landlord, towards the cost of surrendering or reassigning a lease, towards the cost of stamp duty land tax (SDLT).
- PCOs will not cover deficits arising from payment holidays, or borrowings that do not relate to the land purchase, building or extension costs of the old premises.
- Any such payments will be made direct to the lender.
- Business and water rates, sewerage charges and clinical waste removal costs are all reimbursable.
- In certain leased premises service charges are also reimbursed.
- Further guidance notes are provided at www.bma.org.uk on the following areas:
  - Practice premises
  - Service charge agreements
  - Surgery premises: their valuation and an introduction to the rent and rates scheme
  - Cost rent scheme: guidance for GPs
  - Primary care trusts: a guide to estates and facilities matters.

INFORMATION MANAGEMENT AND TECHNOLOGY

- As IM&T systems are replaced PCOs will in future own practices' IT systems and will bear the total capital and maintenance costs.
- GPs are guaranteed a choice of an accredited system and a right to change suppliers every three years.
- PCOs are responsible for training in use of the PCO systems.

- Integration of IT at a community level.
- Issues of confidentiality.
- Practices will have to support requests for new hardware or software with a business case.
- 100% reimbursement of existing systems maintenance.

PERSONAL MEDICAL SERVICES

- The Primary Care Act 1997 introduced PMS.
- This is also a practice-based contract funded through a locally negotiated budget agreed with the PCO.
- The budget is based on the non-discretionary, non-cash limited element of the old GMS contract as a baseline (i.e. including premises funding but not cost rent) uplifted year on year for pay awards and variances in circumstances.
- An element is included for the personally administered or dispensing fees and on costs, maternity cover, prolonged study leave, sickness.
- A PMS practice must have a practice and professional development plan (PPDP).
- In addition, the practice will receive discretionary or cash-limited budgets for practice staff, training, cost rent, improvement grants and computers.
- Some practices may negotiate additional payments for enhanced services.
- The agreed budget is paid in 12 monthly instalments, top sliced for any items paid direct by the PCO, including the estimated superannuation deductions as for GMS.
- PMS practices may take part in the QOF but the maximum points they can achieve is reduced by 105 for 2007/08 because some of the QOF targets are already paid for in the PMS baseline contract figure.
- The main benefit of PMS has been the ability to source growth funding towards additional employment costs of either salaried GPs or nurse practitioners, particularly in under-doctored practices.

PRIVATE FEES

GPs can make charges only in limited circumstances, as follows:
- to statutory bodies for the purposes of that body's statutory function, some of this work will now be classed as NHS work for superannuable purposes, e.g. attendance allowance under special rules
- to employers or schools for routine medical examinations
- for non-primary medical services in a nursing home
- for medico-legal examinations after a road traffic accident
- for attending a police station to examine a detainee
- for medico-legal reports
- for travel immunisations not included in the contract

- for prescribing drugs for foreign travel
- for medical examination for exemption from wearing a seatbelt.

The specific services that a GP can charge his or her own patient for are listed in Schedule 5 of the NHS (GMS Contract) Regulations 2004.

DISPENSING AND PERSONAL ADMINISTRATION

- Where GPs provide personally administered services or provide dispensing services a claim is made for a reimbursement from the Prescription Pricing Authority (PPA).
- The payment is made via the PCO.
- Changes to the payments scheme were introduced for 2006/07 which create savings on VAT and remove incentives to prescribe.
- Some contractors are authorised or required to provide dispensing services to specific patients; the arrangements for this are set out in part 3 of schedule 6 to the 2004 regulations.
- Separate reimbursement arrangements exist for the supply of oxygen and oxygen-therapy equipment.
- Dispensing practitioners are required to charge the patient for the relevant script fee, which is then collected by a deduction at source on the income claim.
- All income and expenditure in respect of dispensing must be shown gross for accounting purposes.

OTHER NHS INCOME

This might include:
- community hospital appointments
- training grants
- PCO/NHS trust appointments.

OTHER REIMBURSEMENTS

These might include:
- registrar's salary and expenses
- towards capital expenditure, e.g. computer hardware, fixtures and equipment, maybe from a PCO incentive scheme, donations, the deanery, remaining fundholding savings or practice-based commissioning savings.

ALTERNATIVE PROVIDER MEDICAL SERVICES (APMS)

- This is intended to offer substantial opportunities for the restructuring of services to offer greater patient choice, improved access and greater responsiveness to the specific needs of the local community.
- It is intended as a tool to address need in areas of under-provision, to enable re-provision of services and to improve areas with GP recruitment and retention problems.
- Guidance for non-GMS contracting arrangements is available on the DoH website.
- PCOs can enter APMS contracts with any individual or organisation that meets the provider conditions as set out in the Directions including the independent sector, voluntary sector, and not-for-profit organisations.
- The focus is on innovation and competition.
- Locally negotiated contract, service specification, performance monitoring.

PRIMARY CARE TRUST MEDICAL SERVICES (PCTMS)

- PCTs are able to provide services themselves by directly employing staff.
- The PCT must comply with the National Health Service Act 2006: PCTMS Directions 2008 and other relevant legislation also published on the DoH website.

LATEST NEWS

There have been no changes to the Carr-Hill formula allocations since the inception of the new contract. Negotiations are expected to commence regarding the 2009/10 contract and in particular the possible removal of the MPIG.

CHAPTER 6

Partners' funds and financing the practice

PARTNERS' FUNDS

The concept of partners' funds is essentially a simple one, but the terminology commonly used can be confusing. The aim of this chapter is to explain what is meant by partners' funds when used in the context of a GP partnership, and why it is important to measure and classify.

The purpose of the balance sheet in the annual accounts is to quantify the value of assets and liabilities at the balance sheet date. The value of the net assets (that is, assets less liabilities) must by definition equal the amount of money the partners have invested in the partnership at that point in time. This value of net assets is what is meant by partners' funds. For a sole practitioner all the net assets belong to him or her. However, in a partnership, the total value of partners' funds must be split so that it is known how much of the total funds invested at any point in time belongs to each partner. When a partner leaves a practice it is their share of the partners' funds that will be repaid to them by the continuing partners.

It is helpful to split partners' funds into two categories: capital accounts and current accounts. Capital accounts are those monies that are invested long term by the partners. In the Upside Medical Practice accounts set out in Chapter 4, the capital account is the difference between the value of the freehold property and the property loan. In addition to this capital representing the equity in the property, some practices also include capital accounts to cover the net book value of fixtures, fittings and equipment, and also working capital. Working capital is usually a round sum invested by the partnership to fund drugs, stock and debtors, that would otherwise have to be funded by bank overdraft. All capital is a long-term investment by the partners and as such is not available to be withdrawn, but is left in the practice until a partner leaves.

Current accounts, on the other hand, represent the difference between a partner's profit share less money withdrawn or otherwise set aside for tax, superannuation or needed for long-term capital. It is good practice after the annual accounts have been approved for each partner to be paid his or her current account balance. This stops inequalities building up where one partner is leaving behind more money than another. It also greatly aids understanding of the accounts if each partner walks away with a cheque each year equal to the balance on his or her current account. The distillation of all the many figures in the annual partnership accounts into one number that a partner can pay into their own bank account concentrates the mind wonderfully! Conversely, if a partner's drawings has exceeded their profit share so that the partner's current account is overdrawn, they will need to pay a cheque into the partnership from their personal resources.

Sometimes there can be confusion between 'current account' in this context of a partner's undrawn profits and 'current account' in the sense of the partnership's bank account and it is important not to confuse the two.

These concepts are easier to understand in the context of a hypothetical example. Drs Y and Z set up a brand new practice on 1 January 2008. They purchase surgery premises for £100,000 and spend a further £25,000 on furniture, fixtures, fittings and equipment. Each doctor puts £15,000 of their own money into a practice bank account, and they take out a loan of £110,000 to finance much of the above capital expenditure. Thus, on day one, the balance sheet of the partnership is as follows.

Balance Sheet at 1 January 2008

Partners' funds	£	£
Capital accounts		
Dr Y	15,000	
Dr Z	15,000	
		30,000
Current accounts		
Dr Y	–	
Dr Z	–	
		–
		30,000
Employment of funds	£	£
Tangible fixed assets		
Surgery premises	100,000	
Furniture, fixtures, fittings and equipment	25,000	
		125,000
Bank loan		(110,000)
		15,000

Current assets	
Bank account	15,000
Net assets	30,000

It can be seen that in addition to providing the funds to purchase the fixed assets, the partners have also paid in an additional £15,000 to cover the working capital requirements of the practice.

The partners decide to pool all income and expenditure and they share the net earnings of the practice equally. The question is: what happens to the partners' funds over the passage of time? Let us assume that the practice buys a computer for £5,000 for which no reimbursement is received. In the above example the tangible fixed assets rise to £20,000 but the practice bank account falls to £10,000. In total the value of net assets remains at £30,000, so the partners' funds must also be £30,000. It follows that the reality of the situation is the partners' funds will only change over time depending on the earnings of the practice compared to each partner's drawings.

Let us now assume that, in the first year ended 31 December 2008, the income less expenses of the practice amounts to £140,000, which is split equally between the partners. The partners have also agreed to meet their own tax liabilities personally. The records of the practice disclose that the partners have taken the following amount in drawings.

	Dr Y	Dr Z	Total
	£	£	£
Monthly drawings	48,000	48,000	96,000
Superannuation contributions	3,498	3,498	6,996
Class 2 NIC contributions	102	102	204
Quarterly special drawings	16,000	12,000	28,000
	67,600	63,600	131,200

Let us also assume that there is no stock of drugs at 31 December 2008 and that all income earned has been received (i.e. no debtors) and all expenditure incurred has been paid (i.e. no creditors) and £2,000 has been paid off the bank loan. Also, the furniture, fixtures, fittings and equipment have been depreciated by £6,000 and this cost has been deducted before arriving at the net earnings of £140,000.

The net assets of the practice at 31 December 2008 will be:

	£	£
Tangible fixed assets		
Surgery premises	100,000	
Furniture, fixtures, fittings and equipment	24,000	
		124,000
Bank loan		(108,000)
		16,000
Current assets		
Bank account		22,800
Net assets		38,800

The partners have decided that the £15,000 working capital they introduced at the outset remains a reasonable figure so the initial partnership capital of £30,000 has increased by £1,000 to £31,000 comprising:

	£	£
Tangible fixed assets		
Surgery premises	100,000	
Furniture, fixtures, fittings and equipment	24,000	
		124,000
Bank loan		(108,000)
Working capital		15,000
Total partnership capital		31,000

This additional £1,000 is not available for the partners to withdraw, so is transferred from their current accounts to their capital accounts.

Partners' capital accounts	*Dr Y*	*Dr Z*	*Total*
	£	£	£
Balance at 1 January 2008	15,000	15,000	30,000
Transfer from current account	500	500	1,000
Balance at 31 December 2008	15,500	15,500	31,000

If the surgery premises had been revalued, any increase (or decrease) in the value would have been added (or deducted) from the partners' capital accounts.

This leaves the partners' current accounts to be prepared. In a nutshell, the formula that always applies to partners' current accounts is as follows.

Current account at the beginning of the period
Add: Share of practice earnings
Deduct: Drawings
Add or deduct: Reduction or increase in partners' capital
Equals: Current account at the end of the period

Using the figures in our example this becomes:

Partners' current accounts	Dr Y	Dr Z	Total
	£	£	£
Balance at 1 January 2008	–	–	–
Profit for the year	70,000	70,000	140,000
Drawings	(67,600)	(63,600)	(131,200)
Transfer to capital account	(500)	(500)	(1,000)
Balance at 31 December 2008	1,900	5,900	7,800

The partners would be advised to withdraw these amounts once the accounts have been approved.

Thus the whole balance sheet at 31 December 2008 becomes:

Partners' funds	£	£
Capital accounts		
Dr Y	15,500	
Dr Z	15,500	
		31,000
Current accounts		
Dr Y	1,900	
Dr Z	5,900	
		7,800
		38,800
Employment of funds	£	£
Tangible fixed assets		
Surgery premises	100,000	
Furniture, fixtures, fittings and equipment	24,000	
		124,000
Bank loan		(108,000)
		16,000

Current assets	
Bank account	22,800
Net assets	38,800

We are now able to define what partners' funds are – they represent the partners' share of the net assets of the practice, being the amount of capital introduced by a partner plus earnings not drawn to date.

FINANCING THE PRACTICE

Having established the concept of partners' funds and the distinction between partners' capital and current accounts, it is useful to look in further detail at the choices to be made when partners consider how they fund their practice.

It would be unusual, but not unknown, for partners to provide all the funds that the practice requires themselves. At the other extreme, partners may provide no capital at all and rely wholly on bank or other borrowing. In reality practices will fall between these two extremes and the characteristics of such practices can be categorised according to the views of the partners.

No bank borrowing/high partners' funds	*High bank borrowing/low partners' funds*
←	→
Aversion to risk	Desire to maximise funds withdrawn from the practice
Partners looking to build up a 'nest egg' to be paid to them on retirement	No anticipation of large payout on retirement
New partners expected to introduce capital, either by initial cash contribution, or by restricting drawings in early years	No requirement for new partners to introduce funds
Regular monthly drawings with annual drawdown of remaining profits	Drawings are maximised with ad hoc payments during the course of the year
Surplus funds held on deposit within the practice	Practice consistently runs a bank overdraft
Like to hold funds 'for a rainy day'	Unforeseen expenditure needs create funding difficulties

There is no right or wrong position on financing, but it can cause conflicts within the partnership if partners hold diametrically opposing views. The 'normal' position, in so far as one can be recommended, would be along the following lines.

- Any surgery premises owned by the practice are funded by a bank loan equivalent to 80% to 100% of the value of those premises.

- The other fixed assets and working capital needs are funded out of the partners' own funds.

A bank overdraft facility is available, but is only utilised at the time of year when funds are at their low point (e.g. leading up to the receipt of the QOF reward money, or after the payment of January tax bills).

Such a position gives a reasonable balance between ensuring a practice does not have to worry about cash flow on a day-to-day basis, while not requiring new partners to introduce large amounts of cash, which can be detrimental to recruitment.

Partnership loans compared with personal loans

When looking at a practice balance sheet it would be natural to assume that a practice with a higher level of partners' funds is somehow wealthier than one with a lower level. However, very often partners will have personal loans which they took out to buy into the partnership that do not appear on the balance sheet. To see the whole picture it is necessary to know whether the partners have any personal borrowing.

In the example above, at 1 January 2008 Drs Y and Z both had capital accounts of £15,000. However, instead of taking out a partnership loan of £110,000, each partner might have introduced £55,000 of their own money. Let us say Dr Y has sufficient personal wealth to pay in £70,000 from his own savings. Dr Z, however, could only fund £15,000 from her savings and took out a personal loan of £55,000 for the balance of her £70,000 capital contribution. Each partner would be showing as having a capital account in the partnership accounts, but once you allow for Dr Z's personal loan of £55,000, her true investment in the partnership is £15,000. This is the same investment as the original example; the only difference is that instead of having a 50% share of a business loan of £110,000, Dr Z has a personal loan of £55,000.

It can be seen that personal loans are more flexible in that they allow partners to borrow different amounts depending on their own personal circumstances. However, it is administratively simpler if borrowing is in the name of the partnership as it avoids having to repay old loans and take out new ones whenever a partner change occurs. This can also save on arrangement and security fees. It may also be possible to negotiate better terms if the borrowing is consolidated with one lender to the whole partnership than would be possible with individual personal loans.

Taxation considerations for practice finance

Any interest incurred by the partnership on its business borrowing is an allowable expense for tax purposes, so the profits on which the partners pay tax are reduced by the amount of interest paid on the partnership loans. If a partner takes out a personal loan and uses the money to buy into a partnership or contribute capital, the partner can claim tax relief on the interest incurred on that loan when preparing his or her annual tax return. Therefore the tax position is essentially equivalent whether business borrowing is within the partnership or personal, although there can be timing differences if the partnership prepares accounts to a date other than 31 March.

The ability of partners to claim tax relief on loans to a partnership can give a partner the opportunity to restructure their personal borrowing to maximise their tax relief.

Take an example where Dr Q has a capital account balance in his partnership of £50,000. He has no personal business borrowing, but does have a mortgage on his own home of £150,000. With the agreement of his partners he withdraws £50,000 from the partnership, thus reducing his capital balance to nil. This money is used to reduce his personal mortgage by £50,000 to £100,000. The next day he takes out a personal business loan for £50,000 and pays this money into the partnership, which brings his capital account back to the original £50,000. The partnership is therefore left in an unchanged position, although it may seek recompense from Dr Q for any temporary overdraft charges caused by the withdrawal of £50,000 for one day. However, Dr Q, instead of having a personal mortgage of £150,000 now has a personal mortgage of £100,000 and a business loan of £50,000. Even allowing for any differential in interest rates, the tax relief of 40% available to a higher rate taxpayer on the business loan interest will result in a significant saving.

SUMMARY

It is important for every partner to have an understanding of how a practice is financed and the interaction between partners' funds and external borrowing. The concept of partners' capital and current accounts is also essential in enabling a partner to read the partnership accounts and know what this means in relation to his or her personal stake in the business.

CHAPTER 7

Other sources of income

In the thriving and successful practice there is a diversity of private work, some-times accounting for up to 50% of practice income, and any practice wanting to maximise profits should certainly be doing some private work. By that, we mean activities outside the scope of general medical services or personal medical services activities.

In the Association of Independent Specialist Medical Accountants survey of 2007, on average 7.7% of total income was generated from sources outside GMS or PMS. This represented, on average, an income of £22,362 per annum for a full-time equivalent GP. Obviously, this is a significant contribution to the earnings of any GP, and provides protection against financial underperformance in GMS or PMS work.

It therefore follows that many GPs undertake 'private' work because the main GMS or PMS contract might fail to bring in the expected financial rewards for several reasons, such as:
- missed quality targets
- local competition from other providers
- limited range of services due to understaffing
- inability to limit workload
- poorly negotiated national and local pay settlements
- desire to abandon out-of-hours work
- under-utilisation of information technology available
- failure to chase up NHS payments
- low level of payments for work done, e.g. treating violent patients.

However, undertaking private work in itself may not be the right answer. The new contract makes the provision of some services a national requirement of every primary care organisation. These services are too under-utilised in some areas to be required by every practice, so specialisation now becomes an alternative to private income sources. Thus, GP specialists can evolve who provide a service to a number of practices with the primary care trust being the effective employer.

Such services provided to a locality might include:
- cardiology, e.g. echocardiography
- elderly care
- diabetes
- palliative medicine
- mental health, e.g. substance misuse
- dermatology
- musculoskeletal
- women and children
- ENT
- homeless/asylum seekers
- procedures, e.g. vasectomy, endoscopy.

Whether this is all more lucrative than private work depends on the locality. Remuneration is normally pitched at a level to make it appealing to well-paid partners, and training is normally provided by the PCO.

PRIVATE WORK AVAILABLE

To make the comparison, we need to consider what private work might be available. By surveying the accounts of GPs on a regular basis, AISMA has collated a list of 100 ways of obtaining private income. The list, of course, is not exhaustive but at least provides a guide as to what might be available, as follows.

- acupuncture sessions
- authorship fees
- bail hostel fees
- benefits agency work
- biopsy clinics
- blue badge examinations
- character references
- committee fees – BMA
- committee fees – GMSC
- committee fees – MDU
- committee fees – RCGP
- coroners' court reports and attendance
- court of protection reports and certificates
- court reports and attendance fees
- cremation fees
- data collection
- deputising income – cooperatives
- deputising income – Healthcall
- deputising income – rotas
- directorships – ambulance trusts
- directorships – cooperatives
- directorships – deputising companies
- drug company – research
- drug company – trials
- hire of rooms – NHS
- hire of rooms – other health professionals
- hospice appointments
- hospital work – NHS bed fund
- hospital work – NHS casualty service
- hospital work – NHS clinical assistant
- hospital work – NHS practitioner
- hospital work – private
- hypnotherapy sessions
- impotency clinics
- independent tribunal service
- insurance reports

- lecturing fees
- life assurance reports
- LMC chair/secretary
- local initiatives – diabetes, smoking, IHD, etc.
- locum work
- Macmillan service
- medical audit advisory group work
- medical research ethics committee
- medicals – government departments
- medicals – health authority
- medicals – local authority
- medico-legal work
- mentoring fees
- minor surgery – excess over GMS
- minor surgery – non GMS
- minor surgery – vasectomies
- monitoring – anticoagulant, methadone, etc.
- NHS Direct fees
- NHS Direct posts
- NHS trust board fees
- NSPCC
- occupational health
- passport counter signature
- PCG/PCT board fees
- PCG/PCT compensatory allowance
- PCG/PCT meeting fees
- pilot licence reports and examinations
- police training centre retainer
- private consultancy work
- private medical examinations and reports
- private prescriptions
- private vaccinations – yellow fever, travel, etc.
- public health appointments
- reports – department of social services
- reports – insurance companies
- reports – solicitors
- retainer – air force
- retainer – airports
- retainer – army
- retainer – commercial
- retainer – industrial
- retainer – local authority
- retainer – navy
- retainer – nursing homes
- retainer – police
- retainer – prison
- retainer – residential homes
- retainer – retail
- retainer – school
- retainer – university
- retainer – young offenders
- review panel – disciplinary
- shotgun licence certificates
- sick notes
- sports – event attendance
- sports – football club doctor
- sports – injury clinics
- sports – rugby football club doctor
- summative assessments
- teaching fees – medical school
- undergraduate training
- visiting medical officer – local authority
- vocational training course organiser
- war pension domestic visits.

ISSUES TO CONSIDER

The question now is how best to diversify? Should a GP specialise or seek private work that appeals? From a financial point of view what the economists call 'opportunity costing' now comes into play. This basically means that by doing the extra work a GP may be unable to do something else, and might run the risk of losing income. The extra work is financially viable only if the overall balance results in an increase in profit. For example, a GP may gain an income from private work but this must be weighed against the cost of, say, employing a locum. The most cost-effective private work is work that can be dovetailed around existing services, such as doing an insurance medical at the end of a surgery.

Given that 'opportunity costing' is a critical issue, the art of delegation (but not abdication) becomes a crucial aspect of profit maximisation. A secretary who can generate reports frees up GP time – maybe two hours per week. Employing extra nursing time to undertake private contracts such as occupational health results in a good return for the practice. The key is to keep partner time to a minimum without abdicating the entire responsibility. However, to delegate effectively, practices must appreciate that the locums, nurses or salaried GPs *must* be appropriately qualified and work to the high standards demanded by the practice.

The AISMA survey identifies that those practices operating under PMS, particularly the early pilots, earn far more than their counterparts under GMS, by up to £16,000 per annum per full-time equivalent GP. One of the reasons for this disparity is that PMS practices had access to growth monies, which paid for the employment of salaried GPs or nurse practitioners. This freed up time for PMS GPs to undertake specialisation supported by the PCOs or private work, all of which resulted in increased profits, provided that the art of delegation was conducted properly and appropriately without loss in patient care overall.

But all that glistens is not gold. There are clear pitfalls in pursuing the route of specialisation or private work. These are broadly summarised as follows.

- Beware the ego trap – flattery, title or status can be nice, but is a GP a better person for simply filling a vacant post?
- Beware escapism – it might appeal to obtain a couple of sessions away from routine surgery work per week, but will it cover the additional costs (e.g. locums), and remember that the paperwork will still await the GP on return to the practice.
- Beware the partners' resentment – losing money to the practice is bound to create resentment. It is best to take on work that earns all of the partners a visible profit.
- Beware compressing existing surgery work into a shorter time – always delegate something else in return and decide how busy as a GP you should be. Letting work mount up is not the way to maximise profit.

When considering work outside GMS or PMS, GPs must be aware that if private work conducted on NHS premises exceeds 10% of total income, the cost rent available to the practice will be reduced. Consequently, if more than 10% of practice income is to be generated by private work, ensure that much of it is conducted 'off site' so that the cost rent is not renegotiated downwards.

The superannuation rules that came into effect on 1 April 2004 provide that the superannuable income of a GP equates to their net profit from the NHS. This net profit is the taxable NHS profit of each and every GP in the UK. Clearly, the private income of a GP, whether retained personally or pooled, becomes part of this calculation. It therefore follows that a GP needs to consider whether private work (i.e. non-GMS or PMS) should be within or outside the NHS, as the former will enhance superannuable income, whereas the latter will only have a pension effect if dealt with through the private pension market.

Another issue that GPs should be aware of is their GMS or PMS contract which provides that GMS or PMS services must be provided by practices from 8 am to 6.30 pm from Monday to Friday. This clearly puts a lifestyle strain on GPs seeking to do outside work to supplement income, and makes the art of delegation more important than ever. Extended practice hours will further enhance the strain.

The subject of private income cannot be left without considering the concept of partnership. In any partnership, the partnership agreement will require a partner to devote sufficient time to their duties within the partnership to enable the practice to prosper and operate effectively. Any partner therefore has duties and obligations to the partnership over and above personal gain. The crucial question now is whether specialisation or private work is for the benefit of the partnership as a whole or the individual GP. In any partnership some GPs may be more financially ambitious than the other GPs. The question is how to keep all of the partners happy.

This is yet another reason why a clear partnership agreement is a necessity. In Chapter 3, the suggested contents of a partnership agreement are set out and they include the duties and obligations of partners, which necessarily include the amount of time to be spent on partnership activities. Most practices adopt the policy of income generated from work performed during practice time belonging to the partnership, and income generated from work performed outside practice time belonging to the individual partner, either privately or by way of a prior share. This may be a fair solution but steps should be taken to ensure that the practice does not suffer from an individual partner overdoing other activities in private time. For example, it is not acceptable that an individual partner should perform excessive out-of-hours work in private time if they are then too tired to undertake normal practice activities in practice time.

Finally, on the concept of partnership, it is never a good thing that partners should keep secrets from one another and nor is it healthy for individual partners to harbour feelings of jealousy. Partners should be upfront with one another and fully accept what is agreed between them. In this way, it will be easier for private income to be channelled through the practice accounts, which is more appropriate for benchmarking purposes, easier to deal with the tax note in the accounts and simpler for the superannuation calculations, as the need to complete form GP Solo will be avoided.

Diversity in general practice can be a good thing – it adds interest, wealth and security. However, for most GPs their main NHS contract will provide most of their earnings. The decision to take on extra work is a difficult one – a GP has to balance financial gain against workload and lifestyle. If a GP is happy with their existing workload, extra work can be taken on only by delegating existing tasks or buying in extra help, and this is clearly a very personal decision. Intelligent and honest assessment should be applied to financial opportunities, as cherry picking invariably produces the best returns.

CHAPTER 8

Practice expenditure

Practice expenditure falls under five main headings: staff costs, medical expenses, premises, administration and finance.

STAFF COSTS

Staff costs comprise not only salaries of administration and nursing staff (including employer's national insurance and 14% employer's superannuation contributions) but also the costs of practice-employed salaried GPs, retainers and those practice-employed GPs on flexible careers schemes. Primary care trust contributions to staff salaries are now subsumed within the overall personal medical services budget or general medical services global sum, and separate funds are also available towards salaried clinical staff by way of growth money (although this may be under threat in future), reimbursements via registrar salary reimbursements, retainer scheme allowances and, in the short term, the flexible career scheme. Regarding the last of these, although no new FCS posts are being created and therefore funding will be limited to existing posts, 50% of an existing flexible careers scheme doctor's salary is reimbursable in the first year, falling to 25% in the second year and 10% in the third and final year. Some practices (or their accountants) prefer to disclose salaried GPs, retainers, registrars and flexible careers schemes GPs as medical expenses – there is no right or wrong approach.

Correct recording of staff salaries is essential to comply with the law and avoid expensive conflict with the HM Revenue and Customs (HMRC). To mitigate any problems, it is worth ensuring that:

- correct tax code numbers are operated for all employees
- all employees' national insurance (NI) numbers are recorded
- the correct tax is paid to the collector of taxes and on time
- forms P9D and P11D have been completed where relevant
- all bonuses in cash or kind have been taxed correctly
- forms P45 are completed correctly

- forms P46 are completed correctly for all staff employed for more than one week
- forms P38a are completed correctly for all casual employees.

MEDICAL EXPENSES

Every practice will incur expenditure of this type, and items falling within this category include drugs and medical supplies. It is important to separate the two so that a close eye can be kept on profit margins when comparing income from reimbursable drugs and appliances with the costs incurred.

Other typical items falling within the medical expenses heading may include medical committee levies, locum costs and deputising costs where the practice has not opted out of out-of-hours work. As stated above, medical expenses could also include the salaries of technical as opposed to administrative staff.

PREMISES EXPENDITURE

All practices will incur premises expenditure, but the nature of such expenditure will vary depending on whether or not it is a surgery-owning practice. If the partners (or at least some of them) own the property, they will incur costs on property insurance and potentially ground rent, as well as mortgage interest (a finance cost).

All practices, whether or not they own the premises themselves, will suffer costs in respect of maintenance and repairs, light and heat, rates, water rates and cleaning.

For those practices that lease their property from a third party, there may be clauses within their lease requiring them to redecorate certain areas every few years. If this is the case, it may be advisable to create a sinking fund, estimating the likely annual charge to the practice rather than leaving it to crystallise every, say, three to five years when the partners within the practice may well have changed or altered their profit-sharing ratios. By doing this, a smoothing of the expenditure over the number of years affected creates a truer picture of year-on-year practice profits, and greater fairness between the partners in terms of sharing those costs is achieved. Sinking-fund provisions are not allowable for tax-deduction purposes, however, and tax relief is instead given in the year in which the cost is incurred. An 'equity adjustment' can be made to take this tax effect into account, normally by way of what is known as a deferred tax account, and the practice accountants can give advice on this.

ADMINISTRATION COSTS

The administration costs of the practice are often much the same as those for any other business. Typically, they include items such as telephone charges, postage, stationery, sundry expenses, accountancy charges and computer expenses.

Whereas PCTs have largely taken over the responsibility for acquiring and maintaining practice computer equipment, some elements are not covered, such as payroll maintenance and computer consumables, and practices will continue to incur such costs.

FINANCE COSTS

If the practice has any business loans, such as loans taken out for the purchase of equipment or introducing new capital into the practice, the associated interest would fall under the finance heading, along with bank charges and overdraft arrangement fees.

In addition, where some or all of the partners own the surgery property and have taken out a mortgage to do so, interest thereon will be reflected as a finance cost. If the property is owned in different ratios to those in which profits are shared, a prior charge should be made to the property-owning partners, although a prior share of any incoming rental income will also need to be made.

PRACTICE EXPENSES OR PERSONAL EXPENSES?

Often, certain classes of expenditure can vary significantly from one GP to the next, creating possible inequity. To maintain equality, the partnership agreement should be clear as to what expenditure should be incurred by the practice and what should be met personally. The table below sets out a suggested solution.

Practice	*Personal*
Medical journals, periodicals, books, etc.	Motor expenses
Practice staff (including NI contributions)	Use of home as surgery/study – a proportion
Staff pension scheme	of:
Registrar costs	— rent
Locum and deputising services fees	— water rates
Staff training	— heat and light
Drugs and dressings	— insurance
Disposable equipment	— repairs and renewals
Drugs for prescribing	— window cleaning
Rent	— security expenses
Rates and water rates	— garden expenses
Health centre service charge	— mortgage interest
Heat and light	Locum and deputising fees
Professional indemnity	Spouse's salary and pension scheme
Property repairs and maintenance	Proportion of home telephone
Cleaning and gardening expenses	Proportion of mobile car phone charge
Security	Medical subscriptions
Fire alarm maintenance	Medical journals, periodicals, etc.
Telephone, fax and paging costs	Laundry and cleaning

(*continued*)

Practice	Personal
Postage, stationery, general books and journals	Conference and course fees
	Sundry out-of-pocket expenses
Registrar's motor expenses allowance	Photographic and video costs (proportion)
Equipment repairs, maintenance and hire	Locum insurance
Computer maintenance and expenses	
Accountancy and legal	
Laundry and cleaning	
General expenses	
Bank and loan interest and charges	
Hire purchase interest and leasing costs	
Insurances	
Medical subscriptions	

Where stated under both 'practice' and 'personal', these items are open to debate.

TAX-ALLOWABLE EXPENDITURE

Under income tax legislation, self-employed individuals can claim tax relief on expenditure, whether incurred and paid for by the business, i.e. practice, or by them personally, provided these costs have been 'wholly and exclusively' incurred in the performance of their duties. Put another way, the costs are tax deductible only when they have been incurred as a direct result of and only because of them being in business.

The following table illustrates the normal taxation treatment of typical expenditure.

Allowable	Disallowable
100% annual investment allowance for small businesses with qualifying purchases of up to £50,000 a year. Expenditure in excess of £50,000 will attract a writing-down allowance (WDA) of 20% (10% for integral building fixtures).	Capital expenditure (unless it qualifies for capital allowances)
	Personal expenditure
	Entertaining
	Expenditure for which a refund is obtained
	Life assurance and sickness premiums
Cost of car (restricted to maximum allowance of £3,000 per annum or 20% written-down value, whichever is lower, and subject to private-use adjustment). However, cars emitting not more than 110g/km CO_2 will attract 100% first year allowance, subject to private-use adjustment. Cars emitting more than 160g/km CO_2 will attract a restricted allowance of just 10% per annum, restricted to a maximum £3,000 and subject to private-use adjustments.	

(continued)

Allowable	*Disallowable*
Motor expenses (subject to private use)	
Spouse's salary	
Subscriptions to a medical society	
Public liability insurance	
Medical and surgical equipment insurance	
Subscriptions for medical journals	
Purchase of medical reference books	
Upkeep, cleaning and replacement of medical equipment	
Locum expenses	
Locum insurance (narrow definition)	
Accountancy fees (excluding fees for preparation of personal tax return)	
Training costs (but not those incurred for private purpose or acquiring new skills)	

CAPITAL EXPENDITURE

The distinction between an expense and capital expenditure can often cause confusion. Capital expenditure represents costs that are not day-to-day running expenses of the practice but instead relate to the acquisition of an asset used in or by the practice. Examples of capital expenditure include:

- cars
- surgery premises
- fixtures and fittings
- fire alarms
- medical equipment
- extensions or improvements to surgery premises
- telephone systems
- furniture – desks, chairs, couches, lamps, filing cabinets.

The tax treatment for capital expenditure is different to that for running expenses of the practice.

No income tax relief is granted for expenditure on the construction, improvement or extension of surgery premises. Instead, capital gains tax relief is available when the premises are eventually sold either in entirety or in part.

Capital allowances (effectively a depreciation allowance, determined by the HMRC) are available at various rates for computer additions, cars and plant and machinery, rather than a straight deduction against income, as would be the case for expenses.

ERECTION, IMPROVEMENT OR EXTENSION OF SURGERY PREMISES

If any improvement grant has been received the GPs may have signed an under-taking that they will not claim tax relief, even on the net expenditure. In all other circumstances, GPs should ensure that the architect provides full details of the breakdown of costs, so that those items that attract capital allowances can be clearly identified – this is known as a 'priced bill of quantities'. The point here is that the contract price will always include a substantial amount of expenditure that qualifies for capital allowances, and a claim is not affected if loan finance is obtained. The more common items subject to a capital allowances claim are:

- free-standing and fitted furniture
- kitchen units
- shelving
- storage and filing systems
- reception counters
- refrigerators and other electrical goods
- sound and educational video equipment
- lifts
- central heating and hot-water systems (including hot but not cold-water pipes)
- ventilation and air-conditioning systems
- alarms and sprinkler systems
- carpets, curtains and curtain tracks
- name plates and signs
- coat hooks
- toilet-roll holders
- security grills and shutters.

THE PERSONAL EXPENSES CLAIM

As seen above, expenditure is tax deductible if incurred wholly and exclusively for the purposes of the business, whether or not that expenditure was incurred by the practice or the GP individually. However, since the introduction of self-assessment in 1996/97, partners have been unable to claim practice expenses through their own personal tax returns.

The mechanism for claiming tax-deductible expenses is that of the partner-ship tax return. Whereas personal expenses do not have to be included in the partnership accounts, if they are subsequently brought into the partnership tax return then the expenditure will be treated for all practicable purposes as if it had been included in the partnership accounts.

The partners must ensure that their personal expenses claims are fully justi-fiable and supported by the appropriate documentation. Clearly, claims should represent bona fide expenditure, but without the supporting paperwork the personal expenses could be challenged and ultimately rejected or much reduced if HMRC ever chose to scrutinise and investigate certain aspects of the partnership or individual's personal tax return. Furthermore it is a legal requirement to keep all supporting paperwork for six years.

Certain items incurred personally for business purposes are readily identifiable and cause no problem. These could include costs such as professional subscriptions where they are not paid for by the practice, locum costs, professional journals, accountancy fees (but not for preparation of personal tax returns which are disallowed for tax purposes) and certain courses and conferences. However, care should be taken, as courses attended to acquire totally new skills are not usually tax deductible, nor are the costs of travel or attendance for spouses or other family members who come along, unless it can be specifically proven that their attendance was necessary.

Some personal expenses can be more complex in that they involve a mixture of business and private expenditure and care is needed to ensure a reasonable approach is adopted in identifying the business element and claiming this only in the personal expenses claim.

Two main categories of expenses are affected by this mixed use:
- use of home and/or home phone
- motor expenses.

In recent years, HMRC has become aware that these expenses are sometimes 'grey areas' and claims have been known to come under considerable scrutiny as a result. Therefore care must be exercised when making a claim.

USE OF HOME

A claim for use of home for seeing patients or for undertaking study, writing up notes or performing research can often be justified. If a room is used regularly for practice purposes, most typically a study, there is an argument for claiming expenditure such as heat and light, rates and insurance on a proportional basis, by reference to either the number of rooms in the house or the floor area. HMRC may request detailed records to support such a claim, possibly even visiting the premises to assess if it is reasonable.

Another consideration is capital gains tax (CGT), which can apply on the sale of business assets. In reality, CGT will apply only where one or more rooms are used exclusively for practice/business purposes. A round sum allowance, however, will not trigger a CGT liability and, provided it is not excessive, is likely to be less contentious. Therefore where the house is not used regularly for seeing patients, but some time is spent working from home, a reasonable 'study allowance' based on the number of hours worked per week at home is generally more acceptable. A typical hourly allowance would be in the region of £1 to £6 per week.

As far as use of home telephone is concerned, again, only the business element is eligible for tax relief. Furthermore, telephone line rental is not allowable unless for a specific business line. Itemised telephone bills can be used to identify the proportion of business calls to the total number of calls to establish the percentage of costs that can be entered on the claim.

MOTOR EXPENSES

It is common practice for partnership deeds to require doctors to have their own cars and that these should be used for visiting patients whether at home, in hospital or in nursing homes. Routine and necessary expenditure on cars is tax deductible so long as it is incurred for business purposes, fully recorded, and all invoices and receipts are kept to support the claim.

Typical expenditure will include:
- petrol and oil
- repairs and servicing
- car washing
- parking fees
- AA and RAC subscriptions
- road fund licence
- insurance premiums
- finance charges (interest only).

Only the business element of the running expenses can be claimed and therefore a mileage log should be kept for a typical month or two. Each time the car is used, the mileage should be recorded along with a note as to whether the trip was for business or personal reasons. At the end of the month, the business miles as a proportion of the total miles should be calculated and it is this proportion that can be applied to the total running expenses of the car. If a second car is used, a second mileage log should also be maintained. It is important to remember that travel from home to work and vice versa is not allowable. Given the scrutiny that personal expenses claims can come under, it is essential that a business mileage log is kept to support motor expenses claims. Even if, for example, a 50% claim is made without the appropriate supporting records, such a claim could be challenged and significantly reduced not only for the current year of claim but potentially for the previous six years as well.

Some GPs prefer to lease a car for use in the practice. However, similar records for business use and running expenses have to be maintained.

If the car is owned by the GP, a 'depreciation' allowance known as a capital allowance, generally currently at 20% (although could vary depending on CO_2 emissions), is available on the purchase price of the car, subject to a maximum of £3,000 per annum. However, this allowance is also subject to a private-use deduction. For example:

Car purchased in year 1 for £16,000   16,000

Capital allowance 20%, restricted to £3,000   (3,000)   (subject to private-use deduction)

Tax written down value at end of year 1	13,000	
Year 2 capital allowance 20%	(2,600)	(subject to private-use deduction)
Tax written down value at end of year 2	£10,400	

If the car is used 40% for business purposes, the capital allowance claim would be £1,200 in year 1 (£3,000 × 40%) and £1,040 in year 2 (£2,600 × 40%).

If a GP leases a car, no capital allowances are available, although the lease costs are claimable. However, these are also subject to a maximum amount based on the value of the car, in much the same way as the capital allowances on an owned car are calculated.

SPOUSES' SALARIES

A GP's spouse can be treated as a practice employee, and salaries and pensions paid to them can be a tax-deductible expense for the GP concerned, provided that the relevant duties are actually performed and payment of the salary is genuinely made. If the GP is a higher-rate tax payer and the spouse a non-tax payer or basic-rate tax payer, tax savings can be made. However, HMRC is aware of this and therefore the payment to the spouse has to be wholly justifiable and made at a commercial rate. For example, if a spouse was paid £25 per hour for answering the phone, this may invite enquiry. Payment of salary to a spouse is also less justifiable these days given that so many GPs have opted out of out-of-hours work and see few (if any) patients at home. Where a genuine situation exists, however, it is important to keep a formal record of the duties for which the spouse is engaged. These may include the following:

- reception cover
- telephone answering and making appointments
- secretarial work
- bookkeeping
- chauffeuring.

Although payments are often made up to the national insurance threshold, care needs to be taken. The rate of pay must always be on a wholly commercial basis rather than purely to reduce the tax liability. Payments should be made regularly at weekly or monthly intervals and subjected to the usual employers' responsibilities regarding PAYE and NIC where applicable. If spouses have other employment, it is probably advisable to put them on the practice payroll to ensure that their PAYE and NIC are calculated correctly. Often pension payments are also made to spouses where a salary can be justified, and this enhances the benefits of this type of arrangement.

EXAMPLE PERSONAL EXPENSES QUESTIONNAIRE

Below is a typical example of a questionnaire that should be completed by the GP and returned to their accountants to enable the accountants to prepare a personal expenses claim on the GP's behalf for ultimate inclusion in the partnership tax return and to enable deduction of the expenses against the GP's share of profits.

NAME: ....

PRACTICE NAME: ....

ACCOUNTING PERIOD: ....

Expenses incurred personally in performance of practice/professional duties

Do you use your house for business purposes? This might include reading, receiving telephone calls, administration, course work, being on call, seeing patients at home, writing, e-mails, Internet research, etc.

If so, please describe how, why and the number of hours you spend per week. (This will enable us to assess an appropriate amount for a reasonable claim on your behalf.)

Duties	Hours spent

Do you employ your spouse? If so, please describe duties, estimate of hours worked per week, and total amount paid during the year. If a pension is also paid, please specify the total amount paid.

Duties	Hours per week	Total paid for year
Pension		

Please confirm the amounts are paid at regular intervals into your spouse's bank account.

Car expenses

Do you use your car for business purposes, such as visiting patients, out-of-hours attendance, attending courses, etc? **NB: Travel from home to the surgery, unless on an out-of-hours call, is NOT allowed to be treated as business mileage.** Please keep records for at least ONE MONTH and complete the boxes below:

Car 1

Make of car		
Model of car and approximate age of car		
Engine size		
One month's business mileage	(miles)	£
One month's total mileage (i.e. business and personal)		

Car 2

Make of car		
Model of car and approximate age of car		
Engine size		
One month's business mileage	(miles)	£
One month's total mileage (i.e. business and personal)		

If you bought a new car or sold your old car during the year, please give details and preferably a copy of the relevant documentation for:
- proceeds/part exchange figure for old car
- cost of new car.

Car expenses (EXCLUDING parking or speeding fines, and clamping fines, which are not tax deductible):

	Car 1 £	Car 2 £
Total petrol costs for the year		
Total servicing and MOT costs for the year		
Parts		
Road tax		
Insurance		
AA/RAC membership		
HP interest/repayments (please provide a copy of the agreement)		
Other – please specify		
Car loan – please specify terms, interest rate, repayments, and an interest certificate from the lender		

Do you use your home telephone for business purposes? If yes, please keep records for ONE MONTH, for business calls and total calls made.

	Line 1		Line 2	
	No. of calls made	Cost of calls made	No. of calls made	Cost of calls made
One month's business calls				
One month's total calls				

	Line 1 £	Line 2 £
Total telephone bills for the year (EXCLUDING rental)		

Professional subscriptions **paid personally** (or treated as drawings if paid through the practice):

Subscription to	Amount
BMA	
MDU/MPS	
GMC	
RCGP	
Others (please specify, including whether incurred for NHS or non-NHS work)	

Other general expenses paid personally:

Description			Amount claimed
Stationery			
Mobile phone: equipment calls rental	Total £	Business use %	
Locum costs paid personally (please also provide dates locum worked if possible)			
Replacement of small items (e.g. medical bag items)			
Books/journals			
Dry cleaning/laundry			
Travel and subsistence, taxis			
Course expenses – please provide details			
Computer consumables			
Other (please provide details)			

Have you **personally** purchased any equipment, such as a computer, other office equipment or medical equipment, which you use in the performance of your duties? Please provide details including your best estimate of business use thereof:

Description of purchase	Estimated business use	Date of purchase	Amount

Interest on qualifying loans

If you own part, or the whole, of the practice premises, or have taken out a loan (or top-up loan) to provide working capital, or acquire other business assets, please provide details, **if paid for personally** (i.e. if *not* a practice loan):

Loan provider	Details/purpose of loan	Amount of interest paid in year

NATIONAL INSURANCE

Contributions applicable to GPs:

- Class 1 is in respect of salaried employments paid by deduction at source subject to a lower earnings threshold.
- Class 2 is in respect of self-employment as a partner or sole practitioner in practice and is paid by direct debit to the National Insurance Contributions Office.
- Class 4 is in respect of self-employment as a partner or sole practitioner in practice paid at the same time as personal income tax at the current rate of 8% on profits between £5,435 and £40,040, plus a further 1% on all earnings above the upper threshold.

National insurance is not a partnership expense but the personal liability of each individual GP. Therefore national insurance contributions of any type should always be charged to the partners' current accounts and effectively treated as a drawing.

Where NIC under all three classes above exceed the maximum amount, repayment of excess contributions can be claimed. Alternatively, where it appears that a GP will pay excess NIC, an application can be made to defer Class 4 and potentially also Class 2 contributions. Following year end, HMRC will review all earnings and the GP may be required to pay any underpayment of their total liability once all calculations have been made.

CHAPTER 9

Practice premises

Historically, GPs have been reimbursed the cost of occupying 'appropriate' premises by the Department of Health, the precise mechanism for that reimbursement depending on circumstances. In broad terms, the scale of the reimbursement was governed principally by the number of doctors working in a practice and the number of patients that it looked after.

COST RENT SCHEME

This scheme was very popular with practices and as a result many are still funded under it. In recent years, funding for new projects has been severely curtailed and it is now very rare for new projects to be funded in this way.

The scheme was available for the following types of project:
- the building of completely new premises
- the acquisition of premises for substantial modification
- the substantial modification of existing practice premises.

A paper exercise was carried out to calculate the expected cost of constructing a surgery of the approved size, taking into account regional variations in construction costs, professional fees and VAT. The value of the land as agreed by the district valuer was then added to the sum to establish a theoretical cost of the project. The actual cost rent payment made was then a percentage of that value, with the percentage based on current interest rates.

Having established the approved cost of the project the actual rate of cost rent payment was then dependent on how the project was actually funded. If a fixed-rate loan was taken out then the rate of cost rent payable to the practice was also fixed at the rate ruling when the project was approved. If, however, a variable-rate loan was taken out, the rate of cost rent paid would also vary as interest rates moved.

There is a key issue for those practices that are in receipt of fixed-rate cost – it is only payable while the loan itself remains at a fixed rate. If the loan is changed to a variable rate loan, or it is repaid, the payment to the practice must also switch to the current variable rate. This can have a significant effect on the amount received, since fixed-rate cost rent payments of 9.5% to 11.5% are not uncommon – however, changing the loan would see that coming down to nearer 6% to 7%.

NOTIONAL RENT

In the past, a practice that owns a surgery could have a valuation carried out every three years by the district valuer to establish whether the current market rent of the surgery was more than either the amount being received under a cost rent scheme or the notional rent value currently being paid. If a practice was receiving cost rent but decided to change to receiving the notional rent value because it was now higher, it had to take care because such a change could happen only once.

As the availability of cost rent funding has dried up in recent years it is now more usual to see practices taking on projects on the strength of notional rent payments from day one.

CHANGES IN LIGHT OF THE NEW GP CONTRACT

Prior to the introduction of the new GP contract, premises funding was outside normal funding streams of primary care trusts and was not affected by other aspects of its finances. That situation changed in England when *The National Health Service (General Medical Services – Premises Costs) (England) Directions 2004* were published.

GUARANTEES FOR FUTURE FUNDING

That document introduced a number of important changes. One of its main effects was to establish that while the funding of existing premises was ring-fenced, any new funding for premises had to come from the PCT's overall budget. This change can be clearly seen by the many caveats in the document – paragraph 31, which relates to the funding of leasehold premises' rental costs, is a typical example:

> Subject to the following provisions of this Part, where –
> (a) a contractor which rents its practice premises makes an application to its PCT for financial assistance towards its rental costs; and –
> (b) in the case of rental costs arising under a lease agreed or varied on or after 1st April 2004, the PCT is satisfied (before the lease is agreed or varied), where appropriate in consultation with the District Valuer, that the terms on which the new or varied lease is to take effect represent value for money, the PCT must consider that application and, in appropriate cases

(having regard, amongst other matters, to the budgetary targets it has set for itself), grant that application.

This clearly demonstrates a major change in the government's attitude to practice premises, since for new developments there is no guarantee that increased funding will be available in the future. Where PCTs' budgets are under severe pressure and they find themselves over budget, it is quite likely that premises reimbursements will not be adequately increased.

FUNDING OF COSTS RELATING TO A DEVELOPMENT
One of the plus points to come out of the new arrangements is that PCTs now have the ability to fund some costs and associated VAT that were not covered by the previous scheme. This includes:
- professional expenses – including architects' and surveyors' fees
- legal costs in connection with the purchase of a site and the construction or refurbishment work
- project management
- legal costs in connection with a lease.

GRANTS RELATING TO MORTGAGE PENALTIES ON RELOCATION
The new arrangements allow a PCT to fund redemption penalties where a practice moves into modern leasehold premises, and indeed to meet mortgage shortfalls in negative-equity situations. While there are a number of detailed points that need to be considered, this provides PCTs with the means to overcome major obstacles to practices relocating.

STAMP DUTY LAND TAX IN RELATION TO LEASED PREMISES
It is now possible for a practice to apply to the PCT for financial assistance to cover the cost of any stamp duty land tax incurred as a consequence of signing a lease to occupy premises. However, it is important to realise that while this and the other flexibilities are now available to PCTs, they are not a right that can be demanded by a practice. In reality they are there to help a PCT overcome obstacles where they want a practice to relocate, rather than simply where a practice decides it would like to move.

ABATEMENT OF PREMISES PAYMENTS
One aspect of premises reimbursement that has not changed is the potential for them to be reduced where a practice uses the premises for non-NHS work. The potential reduction in funding occurs where the income earned from non-NHS sources exceeds 10% of the practice's total income. It is important

to note, however, that it is only non-NHS income earned from the practice premises that is taken into account; anything earned off-site is excluded from the calculation.

Once the percentage of non-NHS income earned from the practice premises exceeds 10% of the total income, then all the premises funding is reduced according to the following table.

Private income percentage	Appropriate abatement percentage
Up to 10%	0
Between 10% and 20%	10
Between 20% and 30%	20
Between 30% and 40%	30
Between 40% and 50%	40
Between 50% and 60%	50
Between 60% and 70%	60
Between 70% and 80%	70
Between 80% and 90%	80
Above 90%	90

Although the potential for abatement has always been there, it has rarely become an issue in practice. Given the greater transparency that the new Superannuation Certificates bring with them, it is possible that practices might be asked the question much more in the future.

IMPACT OF IMPROVEMENT GRANTS

In the past, practices that had premises developed with the assistance of improvement grants were in the enviable position of being able to claim an increased rental value on the whole of the development, despite the fact that the state had funded up to two-thirds of the cost. That position was changed in the new premises directions for contributions of NHS capital made after 18 September 2003. In the case of grants made after that date no notional rent payments are made on that proportion of the development for the first 10 years. It has always been the case that no tax relief can be claimed for any expenditure funded by improvement grants. However, GPs no longer have to sign a declaration to this effect, which has led many commentators to take the view that tax relief can indeed be claimed on the net cost. Clarification is currently being sought from the Department of Health.

CHAPTER 10

NHS Pension Scheme

With the introduction of the new contract on 1 April 2004, the method of calculating superannuable earnings changed. The key features are as follows.

- GPs' pensionable earnings are based on their total NHS profits.
- All NHS income is superannuable.
- Dynamising from 1 April 2004 to 31 March 2008 is based on overall actual increases in GPs' superannuable income.
- Following the NHS Pension Scheme Review (*see* later and Chapter 11), dynamisation rates will be based upon the retail price index (RPI) plus 1.5%.
- The primary care trust remains the 'employer'.

NON-GP PARTNERS

The scheme has been opened to non-GP partners (as whole-time employees) and to some out-of-hours providers and their staff, and the following provisions apply:

- They cannot pension any other NHS employments
- The 'employer' is the host PCT
- The PCT must be notified of estimated pensionable pay so that contributions can be deducted from the monthly general medical services/personal medical services payments
- Pensionable pay is based on share of partnership profits
- An end-of-year certificate must be completed
- They are covered by the NHS Injury Benefit Scheme
- They can opt out by completing form SD502.

SOLE TRADER/PARTNERSHIP PENSIONABLE PAY

Superannuable income under the new contract comprises the following:

- GMS/PMS payments net of expenses

- PCO-administered payments net of expenses
- enhanced services payments net of expenses
- quality payments net of expenses
- premises payments net of expenses
- IM&T payments net of expenses
- dispensing payments net of expenses
- other payments made directly by an NHS employing authority to a GP net of expenses, including out-of-hours, board and advisory work, collaborative work (local authorities, prisons) and practice-based work in educating or in organising education of medical students.

COMPANY PENSIONABLE PAY

A company limited by shares may hold a GMS/PMS or SPMS contract. By definition, any entity may hold an alternative provider medical services (APMS) contract. Provided certain conditions are met, any of these entities, other than a limited liability partnership (LLP), may be an employing authority for NHS pension purposes.

New regulations concerning all pension schemes came into force on 6 April 2006. In December 2006, the Department of Health confirmed that, with effect from 6 April 2006, where a limited company holds a GMS/PMS/SPMS/APMS contract, and that company qualifies as an employing authority, and the eligible shareholder is paid a dividend in respect of NHS income, that dividend will be pensioned in the NHS pension scheme.

Where the shareholder is not a general practitioner, the shareholder must be part of the NHS 'family'; essentially an NHS employee or healthcare professional.

Such eligible shareholders' salaries will also be pensioned:
- a shareholder GP's salary will be pensioned as practitioner earnings, and not as officer earnings
- a shareholder who is a non-GP provider will have their income pensioned as a whole-time employee in the officer scheme but cannot pension more than one post. If they have more than one post, they must choose which one to pension
- *see* 'End-of-year certificate' at the end of this chapter for further details.

RECORD KEEPING

Medical practitioners must be aware of the documents and records to be maintained and completed under the new regime, which broadly consists of the following:
- freelance GP locums earnings are pensionable from April 2001, via forms Locum A and B, but from April 2004 if they do out of hours work they must complete the new SOLO form for this, via forms locum C and D

- GP locum work in GMS/PMS is pensionable from April 2002
- GP locum work in alternative personal medical services (APMS) and out of hours (OOH) is pensionable from April 2004
- pensionable pay for all types of GPs continues to be recorded and submitted to the Pensions Agency electronically or in paper form on SD55s
- mainstream GMS/PMS earnings may also include additional or fringe pay, for example out-of-hours work
- principal GPs can choose to pool their fringe earnings or have them paid individually
- if pooled they fall into the practice calculation
- if taken individually they receive an individual pensions credit by completion of new SOLO forms with the relevant employer
- if pooled the fee agreed must include the employer element which is passed to the PCT as part of the calculation mechanism
- the PCT will produce one SD55/SD86 for all earnings of the GP on receipt of the end-of-year certificate
- SOLO forms and relevant contributions must be submitted monthly by the employer to the host PCT
- if a PCT employs a GP under a formal contract of employment a new assistant practitioner pensionable post is set up via form SS14.

ADMINISTRATION AT PCT LEVEL

Again, in an attempt to keep matters as simple as possible, GPs should note the following issues.

- It is possible for a GP to have four types of pensionable income: practice/pooled, individual/SOLO, locum income and pensionable limited company income.
- From 1 April 2004 the employer contribution increased from 7% to 14%.
- It is stated that the employer contribution will be included in the money a practice receives, i.e. it is built in to the amounts paid via GMS, PMS, QOF, etc.
- The PCT top slices payments on account of the final employer and employee contributions based on estimated final superannuable income.
- Actual pensionable income will not be known until practice accounts have been finalised and all tax returns completed.
- The calculation of NHS superannuation contributions payable will be based on the actual NHS profits of each practice each year and will be allotted to individual partners according to their partnership agreement.

TIERED CONTRIBUTIONS

The NHS Pension Scheme Review resulted in the introduction of a new pension scheme for new entrants to the NHS (see later). The review also introduced new employee contribution rates for all members on a tiered basis dependent upon the level of pensionable earnings, which replaces the previous employee rate of 6%. Features of the new rates include the following.

- The rate to be applied for 2008/09 depends upon what type of member you are, how long you have been a member, what type of earnings you have and the level of those earnings in the relevant basis year.
- The rate is to be applied to the whole of your pensionable earnings, not on a sliding scale.
- The NHS Pensions Agency's Technical Newsletter TN05/2008 contains flowcharts and advice for determining which rate to be used.
- Contribution tiers for 2008/09 are as follows:

Tier	2007/08 pay rates	2006/07 pay rates	2005/06 pay rates	New contribution rates
1	Up to £19,682	Up to £19,165	Up to £18,697	5%
2	£19,683 to £65,002	£19,165 to £63,416	£18,698 to £61,869	6.5%
3	£65,003 to £102,499	£63,417 to £99,999	£61,870 to £97,560	7.5%
4	£102,500 and above	£100,000 and above	£97,561 and above	8.5%

- Arrangements must be made with the PCT to deduct at the appropriate rate for 2008/09.
- The rate applicable for 2008/09 will remain fixed, based upon the appropriate basis year, regardless of whether the actual pensionable pay for 2008/09 may mean a higher or lower tier rate could have applied.
- It is not known for future years whether the fixed-rate system above, based upon pay of an earlier year, or the actual rate determined by the year of pensionable pay will be used.

GP PERFORMERS

These might include:

- salaried GPs who are not principals
- flexible career scheme doctors.

GP RETAINERS

The above are treated differently to GP principals and non-GP partners. They are paid by the practice and the practice has prime documentation in respect of the superannuation paid and deducted.

END-OF-YEAR CERTIFICATE

One certificate is required to be completed in respect of income from each source contract. Consequently, should a GP have income from a partnership with a GMS contract, a sole trade with a PMS contract and a limited company with an APMS contract, three certificates would have to be completed. The documents are complex and follow certain rules as follows.

- A pensions agency certificate will be completed once the company corporation tax return, partnership and personal tax returns have been prepared.
- It is submitted to the PCT and any balancing payment made or overpayment refunded.
- The certificate has to be submitted for PCT approval by 28 February after the tax year end.
- Once checked, the PCT adjusts the GP's contributions record and updates the NHS Pensions Agency record by 31 May.
- The certificate takes into account all taxable earnings linked via the various tax returns, separating out NHS income/expenses from non-NHS income/ expenses.
- For sole traders/partnerships, the calculation follows the tax return so is based on practice accounts years ending in the fiscal year, i.e. 30 June 2008, 30 September 2008, 31 December 2008 or 31 March 2009 for 2008/09.
- Similar to the tax system, this creates a pensions overlap which is recorded on the certificate until a GP ceases or there is a change in year end.
- Overlap pension reflects the amount of income that has been pensioned twice at the outset of the scheme.
- Relief is obtained in the final year for the overlap brought forward.
- In a limited company, as the profits distributed by dividend in one year may, in fact, relate to profits earned in an earlier year where a different proportion of NHS to non-NHS income was earned, a pooling system of pensionable profits is used to ensure that NHS profits are not pensioned twice.

ACCOUNTING AND TAX MATTERS

Tax relief for employee contributions and added years has never been in question, under the old or new contracts. Tax relief is received individually on contributions paid in the tax year, with the contributions posted to drawings or director's loan account in the accounts. The position for GP employer contributions is somewhat more complex, as follows.

- Regulations impose the payment of the employer contribution on the practice.
- The AISMA preferred method of accounting is to record the employer contribution as a practice expense in the accounts on the accruals basis.
- HMRC, however, have issued guidance that the employer contribution

is not a tax-deductible expense for the practice, despite it being the legal responsibility of the practice to pay it.

- From 6 April 2006, relief for all pension contributions is now covered by the provisions of sections 188–201 of the Finance Act 2004.
- Section 196(2)(b) provides for tax relief for contributions paid by an employer to a registered pension scheme. However, the NHS Pension Scheme regulations make it clear that, for a GP, the 'employer' continues to be the PCT. Relief is not therefore available under that section.
- The employer contribution is to be viewed as the GP's personal contribution and relief obtained on the tax return for contributions paid in the tax year.
- For periods up to 5 April 2006, HMRC exercised their discretion under Extra Statutory Concession A9 to prescribe that an amount greater than 15% of pensionable pay could receive relief in any one tax year. This enabled relief to be obtained not only on employers, employees and added years contributions paid in the year, but also any arrears of contributions for earlier years paid in a subsequent year.
- After 5 April 2006, tax relief may be obtained on up to 100% of one's relevant earnings. Receiving relief personally for all pension contributions, for whichever year they relate, should not therefore be an issue.

NHS PENSIONS REVIEW

This is covered in detail in Chapter 11, but by way of summary the NHS superannuation scheme will be affected as follows.

- The NHS Pensions Review resulted in a new pension scheme for new entrants to the NHS after 1 April 2008.
- Members of the existing scheme at that time will continue to accrue benefits in the old scheme, with some additional benefits and flexibilities.
- In the new scheme, minimum pension age is 55, with an increased age of retirement without actuarial reduction now 65.
- GPs will be able to draw down part of their pension while continuing to work and contribute to the scheme.
- GPs who joined the scheme after 1 June 1989 (or had a career break from the NHS of 12 months or more after that time) had their pensionable pay capped at a level prescribed annually by the Secretary of State. This cap on the maximum amount of pensionable pay has been removed from 1 April 2008.
- The ability to buy added years service has been removed for both old and new scheme, but members are able to purchase extra pension, even if they have an existing added years arrangement, which itself can continue.
- Added-years contracts in existence at 31 March 2008 will continue to be honoured.
- A notional capping level will continue to apply for members who have

an existing added-years contract at 31 March 2008. So, while the headline employee rate applicable to you will be charged on your total pensionable pay if it is above the cap, your added-years rate will only be applied to the notionally capped income.
- Changes have been made to survivor benefits, death in service benefits and ill-health retirement benefits for both new and old schemes.

GENERAL PENSIONS LEGISLATION

New pension legislation came into effect from 6 April 2006 that affected all schemes. Among the features of the new regulations are the following.
- An upper limit, the Lifetime Allowance (LTA), of pension capital value that may be accumulated (currently £1,650,000 for 2008/09, £1,750,000 for 2009/10 and £1,800,000 in 2010/11).
- Should a value above the LTA be accumulated, the excess may be taxed at up to 55%.
- Protection may be obtained from HMRC against such charges if one's pension 'pot' at 5 April 2006 was already above the LTA set for 2006/07, or was below the LTA at 5 April 2006, but rises above it at retirement within certain parameters. HMRC form APSS200 should be completed and forwarded to HMRC by 5 April 2009.
- In addition to the LTA, there is also a maximum Annual Allowance. This is the maximum by which an individual's pension rights may increase in one year. Increases in excess of this are chargeable at 40%. The Annual Allowance for 2008/09 is £235,000, £245,000 for 2009/10 and £255,000 in 2010/11.

APPENDICES

Example 2007/08 Sole Trade/Partnership Pension Certificate – this is the draft version as submitted to the NHS Pensions Agency and, at the time of going to press, was awaiting Department of Health approval.

GP (and non GP) Providers Annual Certificate of Pensionable Profits 2007/08

To be completed by all GMS, PMS, SPMS and APMS GP (and non-GP) Providers who are partners or 'single-handers'

NOT to be completed where the Practice is a limited company, or by any Salaried GPs.

		Box
Provider's full name		A
Type of contract (ie GMS, PMS, SPMS, APMS) that this Certificate refers to.		B
NI number or Pension Scheme Ref No		C
Practice Reference Number **and** Scheme Employing Authority code		D
Host PCT/LHB		E
Practice accounts year end, to which this Certificate relates (e.g. 30.06.2007, 31.03.2008)		F
GP Private fee (self employed) accounts year end, where private fees are not fed through the Practice accounts (e.g. 30.06.2007, 31.03.2008)		G
Tax and NHS Pension Scheme year end, which the profits at Box 38 relate to (enter NHSPS date)	31/03/08	H
Enter **'Yes'** if earnings cap applies, otherwise leave blank		I
Enter 'Yes' in this box if figures in this Certificate are from a provisional tax return		J

All entries on this form should be completed with reference to all income and expenditure in respect of the GP or non GP Provider

Please refer to the guidance notes when completing this Certificate

Calculation of GP share, or non-GP share of total NHS income and non-NHS income, for the expenses ratio

			Box No.
Step 1	Specify your GP (or non-GP) share of income declared in boxes 3.29 & 3.50 of the full practice partnership tax return of your medical practice, adjusted for tax purposes (i.e. reflects your share of boxes 3.29 and 3.50 minus your share of box 3.71).		1
Step 2	Add your self employed income declared in boxes 14 & 15 of the self-employment (full) pages of your tax return, in respect of medical related work, adjusted for tax purposes (i.e. reflects boxes 14 plus 15 minus 60) Use box 8, 9 & 27 where income is below £64,000 on the 'short' pages	+	2
Step 3	Add your medical related employed income reflected in box 1 of the employment pages of your tax return.	+	3
Step 4	Add your other medical related income, before expenses, declared elsewhere on your tax return, adjusted for tax purposes.	+	4
Step 5	Deduct your income included above in Boxes 1, 2, 3 and 4 pensioned separately	-	5
This is your total medical NHS & non-NHS income for the purposes of the income ratio		=	6

Turn to Page 2

Calculation of GP (or non- GP) share of total non-NHS medical income for the expenses ratio Box No.

Step 1   State the amount of income included in Box 1 above
relating to non NHS income   [   ]   7

Step 2   State the amount of income included in Box 2 above
relating to non NHS income   +   [   ]   8

Step 3   State the amount of income included in Box 3 above
relating to non NHS income   +   [   ]   9

Step 4   State the amount of income included in Box 4 above
relating to non NHS income   +   [   ]   10

Step 5   Deduct your income included above in Boxes 7, 8, 9 and 10
pensioned separately   -   [   ]   11

This is your total non-NHS income for the purposes of the income ratio   =   [-]   12

Calculation of non-NHS income: Total medical income ratio   Box No.

Step 1   Divide Box 12   [-]   Total non-NHS Income   =   [   ]   13
         By Box 6   [-]   Total NHS and non-NHS income   #DIV/0! %

Calculation of total expenses

Step 1   Specify the total of your GP or non-GP share of expenses declared in boxes
3.46, 3.48 & 3.64 of the full practice partnership tax return, in respect of medical related
work, adjusted for tax purposes (i.e. reflects the total of your share of boxes 3.46, 3.48 & 3.64
minus your share of box 3.69 plus your share of box 3.70).   [   ]   14

Step 2   Add the total of your self employed expenses declared in boxes 30
of the self-employment (full) pages of your tax return, in respect of medical
related work, adjusted for tax purposes (i.e. reflects the total of boxes 30
& 55 minus box 59).
Use box 19 plus 22 minus boxes 23 & 24 where income is below £64,000
on the self employment (short) pages.   +   [   ]   15

Step 3   Add your employed expenses declared in boxes
17, 18, 19 & 20 of the employment pages of your tax return
in respect of medical related income   +   [   ]   16

Step 4   Add your medical related expenses claimed elsewhere
or set against income declared elsewhere on your tax return +   [   ]   17

Step 5   Add interest paid on a loan for professional purposes
not accounted for in boxes 14 to 17   +   [   ]   18

This is your total expenses in application of the income ratio   =   [-]   19

Turn to Page 3

Calculation of Pensionable Profits

Box No.

Taxable profit from practice partnership	**(Box 1 - Box 14)**		20
Taxable profit from self employment pages	**(Box 2 - Box 15)**	+	21
Taxable employed income less related expenses	**(Box 3 - Box 16)**	+	22
Other medical related income declared on tax return	**(Box 4 - Box 17)**	+	23
Total of boxes 20 to 23			24
Less: Your interest paid (Box 18)		-	25
Less Any amount included in boxes 20 to 23 pensioned separately (see note 26 particularly regarding pooled salaried appointments. Do **not** include GP SOLO income here)		-	26
Less Your total non-NHS income (Box 12)		-	27
Add Any other pensionable NHS GP income NOT in boxes 20 to 23 that has not been pensioned separately		+	28
Add Your non NHS expenses (Box 61, 67 or from Box 68 under your own method)		+	29 #DIV/0!

If you have not used the standard method of apportioning non-NHS expenses tick this box and enter your explanation in the box 68. 30

N.B. USING THE ALTERNATIVE OR YOUR OWN METHOD OF CALCULATING NON-NHS EXPENSES CAN AFFECT THE LEVEL OF YOUR SUPERANNUABLE PRACTITIONER PAY. NHSPA CANNOT OFFER ADVICE ON WHICH METHOD MAY BE MOST APPLICABLE OR BENEFICIAL TO YOU. PROFESSIONAL ADVICE MUST BE SOUGHT FROM YOUR ACCOUNTANT OR INDEPENDENT FINANCIAL ADVISER SHOULD YOU REQUIRE IT.

		=	31 #DIV/0!
Less: GP SOLO income included above for the accounting year of the SOLO income		-	32
		=	33 #DIV/0!
Multiply Box 33 by the fraction	#DIV/0! x $\frac{100}{114}$	=	34 #DIV/0!
Add: GP SOLO income entered in box 32		+	35
		=	36 #DIV/0!

Memo Pension overlap profits brought forward		37a	
Add: Pension overlap generated in the year		37b	
Less: Deduct pension overlap profits used this year		-	37
Memo Pension overlap profits carried forward or set back against previous years income	-	37c	

This is your Pensionable profit = 38 #DIV/0!

Memo Enter the amount of **SENIORITY** allocated to you per the practice accounts 38a

Amount of Pension Cap for the Year (where this is below the published amount because of income pensioned elsewhere, please provide details at Box 68) 39 112,800

Turn to Page 4

Calculation of NHS Pension Scheme Contributions

	Relevant %		Amount in box 38 or 39 multiplied by % stated in boxes 40 to 43 is contributions due		Contributions already paid and recorded by the PCT/LHB for 2007/08 in respect of practice income		Contributions already paid and recorded by the PCT/LHB for 2007/08 in respect of GP SOLO income		Contribution due less contributions paid	Box No.
Employee pension contributions	6%	40	#DIV/0!	44		48		52 =	#DIV/0!	56
Added years pension contributions*	0.00%	41	#DIV/0!	45		49		53 =	#DIV/0!	57
Money Purchase AVC* contributions	% £	42 42a	-	46		50		54 =	-	58
Employer pension contributions	14%	43	#DIV/0!	47		51		55 =	#DIV/0!	59

Total amount of contributions (over)/under paid for the year   #DIV/0!   60

* You must enter zero or the actual %

Calculation of non-NHS expenses

If the standard method shown cannot be used, the alternative method shown must be used.

Where the GP, or non-GP is required to use the alternative method, accounting records will need to be amended to record this information adequately on an item by item basis.

The standard method for the calculation of non-NHS expenses:

Divide Non-NHS income (Box 12)   _____ -   x Expenses (Box 19)   -   =   #DIV/0!   61
By total income (Box 6)   -

The alternative method for the calculation of non-NHS expenses:

Take the total expenses shown in Box 19   -   62

Less   Expenses wholly attributable to NHS income   -   63

Less   Expenses wholly attributable to non-NHS income   -   64

Expenses that cannot be separately allocated to NHS   =   65
or non-NHS income   -

Ratio for allocation of expenses not separately allocated:

Divide Non-NHS income (Box 12)   _____ 0.00   x (Box 65)   -   =   #DIV/0!   66
By total income (Box 6)   0.00   expenses

Total non-NHS expenses   66   #DIV/0!   +   64   -   =   #DIV/0!   67

Or your own method

If the above calculation and allocation ratio does not give you a fair conclusion, you must use an alternative method of your own, and clearly explain your reasons and methodology in the box provided on page 5 (Box 68).

Turn to Page 5

If you cannot use the standard or alternative non-NHS expense calculations explain your own method of non-NHS expense calculation here:

Box No.

68

GP Declaration

Now you must read and sign the statement below and send this completed Certificate to the appropriate PCT/LHB as soon as possible and NO LATER THAN 28th February 2009 If you give false information you may be liable to prosecution.

"I confirm that information provided on this Certificate is correct and is consistent with my HMRC tax return. I also confirm that my declared NHS pensionable pay does not include any non NHS (i.e. private) income.

GP (or non-GP)   .   Date
Provider's signature

An electronic spreadsheet version of the Certificate is acceptable subject to a paper page 5 being provided with the Provider's signature.

PCT/LHB Agreement

I have checked the figures shown in boxes 38 and 39 of this Certificate and am satisfied that they appear consistent with the relevant NHS work and income that this PCT/LHB is aware of and confirm that they have been used to confirm, record and pay over to the NHS Pensions Division the appropriate NHS Pension Scheme contributions for the year to which this Certificate relates.

PCT/LHB authorised signature   Date

(To be signed by the host PCT at the end of the Provider's contract where it ceases before year end or at 31 March 2008 where the appointment has been throughout the year - see notes to Boxes C and D)

Provider's name

0

NI number or Pension Scheme Ref No

0

Practice Reference Number (see note D)

0

Pensionable profit

#DIV/0!

(The pensionable profit is the amount to be declared on the SD55; i.e. the amount in box 38 or 39)

Example 2007/08 Limited Company Pension Certificate – this is the draft version as submitted to the NHS Pensions Agency and, at the time of going to press, was awaiting Department of Health approval.

GP Provider (or non-GP Provider) Shareholder of a qualifying Limited Company Certificate of Pensionable Income for 2007/08

To be completed by all GP (and non-GP) providers who are shareholders in a limited company that holds a GMS, PMS, APMS or SPMS contract and is a Scheme Employing Authority

The main 2007/08 Certificate may also need to be completed if not all of your pensionable earnings derive from this one company contract.

NOT to be completed by a salaried GP employed by a limited company who is not a shareholder.

Provider's full name		A
Provider's NI number or Pension Scheme Ref No		B
Company's full name		C
Company's employing authority code		D
Company's registered number		E
Type of contract; i.e. GMS, PMS, APMS, SPMS, etc.		F
Host PCT/LHB		G
Company accounts year end falling in the tax year (e.g. 30.06.07, 31.03.08)		H
Tax and NHS Pension Scheme year end, to which the pensionable income at box 13 relate.	31-Mar-08	I
Enter 'YES' if earnings cap applies		J
Tick this box if figures in this certificate are from a provisional return		K

Please refer to the 'Limited Company Guidance And Completion Notes' when completing this Schedule

Calculation of the company's NHS income ratio

Box No.

Step 1 State the company's total NHS and non-NHS income (adjusted for tax purposes) **excluding** shareholders' income that has been pensioned separately.   1

Step 2 State the amount of income included in Box 1 above relating to non-NHS income.   2

Step 3 Deduct the non-NHS income stated in Box 2 from the income stated in Box 1. =   3
This is the company's total NHS income.   -

Calculation of NHS income: total income ratio

Step 1 Divide Box 3   -   Total NHS Income   =   4
By Box 1   -   Total NHS and non-NHS income   #DIV/0!

Turn to Page 2

Calculation of pensionable profits drawn down as a salary   Box No.

Step 1   Enter your gross salary from the company to which this Certificate relates for the tax year,   5
per box 1 of the Employment page E1 your personal tax return. This must be net of any
employment expenses claimed on your tax return.

Step 2   Multiply the figure in box 5 by the figure in Box 4   =   6
This is your gross NHS pensionable salary   #DIV/0!

Calculation of pensionable profits drawn down as dividends

Step 1   Total **net** dividends paid to you in the tax year by the company to which this Certificate   7
relates, per box 3 of page TR3 of your tax return.

Step 2   Multiply the figure in Box 7 by the figure in Box 4   8
This results in your net dividends in respect of NHS income.   #DIV/0!

Step 4   Enter the figure in Box 42, if negative; this is the restriction of the pensionable   9
dividends to profits earned from the NHS.   #DIV/0!

Step 5   Deduct the figure in Box 9 from the figure in Box 8; this is your NHS   =   10
pensionable dividends.   #DIV/0!

NHS pensionable pay

Step 1   Add the figures in Boxes 6 and 10 together and enter the total in Box 11.   =   11
#DIV/0!

Step 2   Enter the gross amount of any outside salaried appointment in your name paid into   12
the company, and pooled with other income, that has already been pensioned

Step 3   Deduct box 12 from box x 11.   This is your pensionable income for 07/08   8   13
#DIV/0!

Memo   Amount of pension cap for the year (where this is below the published amount because   14
of income pensioned separately, please provide details in box 43)

Memo   Enter your provisional SENIORITY entitlement per the company accounts   15

Turn to page 3

Calculation of NHS Pension Scheme Contributions

	Relevant %	Amount in box 13 multiplied by % stated in boxes 16 to 19 is contributions due	Contributions already paid and recorded by the PCT for 2007/08 in respect of company income	Contributions deducted in error from shareholder's salary from the company to which this Certificate relates; training grants, pooled OOH etc		Contribution due less contributions paid	Box No.
Employee pension contributions	6% `16`	#DIV/0! `20`	`24`	`28`	=	#DIV/0! `32`	
Added years pension contributions	0.00% `17`	#DIV/0! `21`	`25`	`29`	=	#DIV/0! `33`	
Money Purchase AVC contributions	0.00% `18` £ `18a`	#DIV/0! `22`	`26`	`30`	=	#DIV/0! `34`	
Employer pension contributions	14% `19`	#DIV/0! `23`	`27`	`31`	=	#DIV/0! `35`	

Total amount of contributions (over)/under paid for the year   #DIV/0! `36`

Calculation of pensionable profits pool

Step 1 Enter your brought forward undistrubted pensionable profits figure, if positive, from box 42 of your previous years limited company schedule.   `37`

Step 2 Enter your theorectical share of the profit after tax but before dividends earned in respect of the accounting year ending in the tax year to 5 April 2008, based upon the ratio indicated in the guidance notes to this box   `38`

Step 3 Multiply the figure in Box 38 by the figure in Box 4 This is your share of potential pensionable profits   = #DIV/0! `39`

Step 4 Enter the figure from Box 8.   #DIV/0! `40`

Step 5 Deduct the figure in Box 40 from the figure in Box 39 This is your current year undistributed pensionable profit   = #DIV/0! `41`

Step 6 Add box 37 to box 41 This is your total undistributed pensionable profit carried forward. (See below if this figure is negative)   #DIV/0! `42`

If the figure in Box 42 is negative, it should be entered in Box 9.

Additional explanatory information, if required   `43`

Turn to page 4

DECLARATION

Now you must read and sign the statement below and send this completed Certificate to the appropriate PCT/LHB as soon as possible.

If you give false information you may be liable for prosecution.

"I confirm that the information provided on this Certificate is correct and is consistent with my HMRC tax return. I also confirm that my declared NHS pensionable pay in Box 13 does not include any non-NHS (i.e. private) income or NHS income pensioned elsewhere."

GP (or non-GP)
Provider signature _____ Date _____

An electronic spreadsheet version of the Certificate is acceptable subject to a paper page 4 being provided with the Provider's signature.

PCT/LHB Agreement

I have checked the figures shown in boxes 13, 14 and 15 of this Certificate and am satisfied that they appear consistent with the relevant NHS work and income that this PCT/LHB is aware of and confirm that they have been used to confirm, record and pay over to the NHS Pensions Division the appropriate NHS Pension Scheme Contributions for the year to which this Certificate relates.

PCT/LHB authorised signature _____ Date _____

(To be signed by the host PCT/LHB at the end of the Provider's contract where that contract ceases before year end or at 31 March 2008 where the contract has been throughout the year).

Provider's name	#VALUE!
NI number or Pension Scheme Reference number	#VALUE!
Company's full name	#VALUE!
Company's NHSPS Emploing Authority Code	#VALUE!
Pensionable profit	#VALUE!

(The pensionable profit is the amount to be declared on the SD55; i.e the amount in box 13 or 14)

CHAPTER 11

Pensions and personal financial planning

As explained in Chapter 10, GPs contribute to the NHS Superannuation Scheme on the basis of their NHS profit, but there are further considerations to take into account, not least of which are the methods of enhancing benefits.

ADDED YEARS

GPs have the option, normally exercised on their birthday, to enhance their pension benefits by the purchase of added years. They pay a fixed percentage of their superannuable income, based upon their age next birthday and the amount of years they wish to purchase, and this will provide enhanced benefits in the shape of extra pension and lump sum at their chosen retirement date. Added years also improve any ill-health early retirement pension and dependants' death-in-service pensions. Taken together, total service plus added years must not exceed 40 years at age 60. The maximum amount of added years that can be purchased is limited to 9% of superannuable remuneration, or the maximum to reach 40 years' service (at 60). Occupational schemes limited 'employee' contributions to 15% of pay, and as GPs paid 6% in the past, the maximum extra payment was 9%. New pension legislation abolished these limits from 6 April 2006. The NHS, however, irrespective of the actual main contribution made by a GP, has decided to retain the 9% limit.

The existing added-years contract is now being replaced, but members who have expressed an interest, before 31 March 2008, have until 31 March 2009 to exercise that interest. Under the new added-years contract GPs buy multiples of £250 up to a maximum of £5,000 extra pension. HMRC limit tax relief on pension contributions up to 100% of UK earnings in one financial year. If GPs pay over this, no tax relief is allowed. Unlike old added-years contracts which automatically included dependants' pensions, GPs now have the choice to decide what if any extra dependants' pension they buy. The new contract does not automatically include a lump sum at retirement.

If GPs can purchase an old-style added-years contract before 31 March 2009, this should be done. If they cannot, our preferred option is to use the new added-years contract before contributing to any other money purchase alternative. Independent advice should be sought.

UNREDUCED LUMP SUM

Those GPs who were members of the NHS Pension Scheme prior to March 1972 will receive a lump-sum retiring allowance for each year of service prior to that date at one-third of the rate applicable to each year afterwards. GPs are able to make up the missing proportion of the lump sum subject to similar conditions applicable to the purchase of added years.

AVCS/FSAVCS

Additional voluntary contributions/free-standing additional voluntary contributions also provide a method for enhancing pension benefits. The key points to remember are as follows.

- AVCs/FSAVCs are 'bolt on' pension contracts supplied through insurance companies that will offer the GP a pension income in retirement dependent on investment growth/annuity rates applicable at the time. The designated AVC suppliers for the NHS are Standard Life and Clerical & Medical.
- A number of insurance companies offer 'free-standing' AVCs, although these are not sold as often nowadays since the introduction of stakeholder pensions.
- AVCs/FSAVCs offer an option where added years prove too expensive to purchase for older GPs.
- Contribution limits are now higher than for added years, but unlike added years AVCs and FSAVCs:
  - are not protected in the event of ill-health early retirement.
  - do not have ancillary benefits included automatically in added years, such as indexation and spouse's/dependant's pensions, unless purchased at the time of drawing the pension, this having the effect of reducing the income supplied. However, it must be stressed that added years once contracted into can only be stopped due to extreme financial hardship, whereas free-standing AVCs can be reduced or stopped in these circumstances.

STAKEHOLDER PENSIONS/SELF-INVESTED PERSONAL PENSIONS

Under stakeholder rules anyone can invest up to £3,600 per annum and attract tax relief on the contribution subject to not breaching the maximum limits. This in essence is 100% of Schedule E/D income in any one tax year. These arrangements have an effective 1% annual management charge and they do limit investment choices.

For GPs wanting to make larger payments who wish to exercise a degree of control over their investment strategy then a self-invested personal pension (SIPP) may be appropriate. A SIPP is more expensive than a stakeholder pension, but there is a good deal more investment freedom and flexibility. If the right advice is obtained, this option should provide better returns in the long term.

'A' DAY

In April 2006 the current eight different pension regimes were replaced by just one. This is based upon a lifetime allowance (initially set at £1.5 million). Occupational schemes such as the NHS scheme are included within this funding limit. A tax-recovery charge of 55% will be levied on funds breaching the allowance. A member's contributions will now be limited to 100% of their income up to a maximum of £215,000 per annum initially. Occupational schemes may elect to keep their scheme rules intact and it is likely that many, due to the potential administrative nightmare involved, will do so. Finally, up to 25% of the pension 'pot' may be taken tax free. The NHS has now adopted this rule. If GPs elect for the higher payment, they need an investment return of 8.33% per year index linked with inflation to cover the lost income. It does not affect the dependant's pension. Independent advice should be obtained before making this decision.

The 'A'-Day limits are as noted below. It is possible to protect against this recovery charge if GPs are above the limits of 5 April 2006. This is done by multiplying the annual pension at the date by 20 and adding on the lump-sum payment. GPs have until 5 April 2009 to register this protection. Do not confuse the 'A'-Day limit with dynamised earnings; they are two different things.

Lifetime allowance	Annual allowance
£1.5 in April 2006	£215,000 in April 2006
£1.6 in April 2007	£225,000 in April 2007
£1.65 in April 2008	£235,000 in April 2008
£1.75 in April 2009	£245,000 in April 2009
£1.8 in April 2010	£255,000 in April 2010

The above annual contribution limits also take into account the 'value' of employer's contribution. If you are a high-earning GP, extra care needs to be taken and specialist advice should be sought.

NHS PENSION REVIEW

Members who joined prior to 1 April 2008 will retain the old-scheme rules and a retirement age of 60. The pension will still be based upon 1.4% of dynamised earnings and 4.2% is the tax-free lump sum. GPs now have the option of taking

25% of their 'pot' tax free. The earnings cap has also been removed so now all earnings will be pensionable for those who joined after 1 June 1988.

New members of the scheme will have a retirement age of 65 and the pension will be 1.87% of dynamised earnings. The lump sum will be by commutation and GPs will get £12 cash for each £1 of pension given up.

The earliest retirement age will increase to 55 from 6 April 2010 for all members. The same early retirement penalties will be applied to both arrangements.

ILL-HEALTH EARLY RETIREMENT

The scheme changed from 1 April 2008. There is now a Tier 1 Pension and a Tier 2 Pension.

Tier 1 Pension

If you are assessed as being permanently incapable of doing your own job, you will be entitled to the early payment of the retirement benefits you have earned to date without any penalty.

Tier 2 Pension

If you are assessed as being permanently incapable of engaging in regular employment of like duration, you will be entitled to the retirement benefits you have earned to date enhanced by two-thirds of your prospective membership up to your normal retirement date.

PERSONAL INSURANCE

It may be appropriate for a GP to consider a number of personal insurances to safeguard current income and future earnings. The following outlines the more common forms of cover often sought by GPs.

Locum cover

This will produce a monthly income to allow a partner absent from work to fund for a locum replacement. This will enable the partner to continue to take regular drawings from the practice. Premiums enjoy tax relief and the policy should mirror the stipulations of the partnership agreement. Consideration should be given as to whether the primary care trust will allow any locum reimbursement when the level of cover is set. Care should be taken when selecting a contract and advice sought, as many of the policies on the market at the present time are general insurance contracts which are reviewable annually, may well not allow multiple claims, and can be cancelled by the insurer at any time.

Income protection

An income-protection contract will supply a tax-free income payable to a GP on the cessation of locum cover once the partnership has come to an end. The maximum income allowable is a percentage of the GP's gross remuneration. Premiums do not attract tax relief but the income is tax free in payment and paid up to the client's selected retirement age. It may be level or escalating. Permanent health insurance contracts cannot be cancelled by the insurer and will allow for multiple claims. Premiums may be guaranteed or reviewable (the latter only in light of overall claims experience). Older GPs may wish to take into account ill-health retirement pension benefits when calculating their income requirements.

Critical illness cover

This is a relatively new form of protection covering severe illnesses (heart attack/ stroke/cancer) which are survived. This type of policy can produce a lump-sum or income-based benefit and is used for a number of purposes, typically:
- to cover loans/mortgages
- to enhance shortfall pension benefits
- to provide for schools fee planning/child care costs
- to enable a partner to either reduce their hours or take time away from work
- for modifications to private dwelling (in the event of severe disablement) or help towards the purchase of a new property
- for long-term nursing care.

Premature death (life cover)

These types of policy are used to pay loans, to replace income, or to fund for an event, or, in the case of inheritance tax, to pay a tax bill in the future (i.e. on second death). The life cover could be for personal or business protection and can be paid out in the form of a lump sum or as regular income over a fixed term. The premiums are relatively inexpensive. Trusts could be considered for any life assurance contract as they have the effect of removing the benefit from the donor's estate and thereby avoid inheritance tax. Life cover can be added, often at minimal cost, to critical-illness contracts.

Endowment policies

Many GPs held endowment plans securing their practice or residential loan(s). In light of recent falling stock markets it is wise to review the situation and check if there is likely to be a shortfall on the policy. The options are as follows.
- Do nothing and hope growth rates pick up.
- Pay more money into the endowment plan.
- Save elsewhere towards a shortfall (ISA/bank accounts).
- Pay more into the mortgage loan itself – either by converting part of the loan into a repayment mortgage or, if the loan is set on a flexible basis, increasing the payment to the lender, thereby reducing the capital balance.
- Surrender the policy, pay off part of the loan with the proceeds and convert the rest to a repayment (capital and interest) mortgage.

- Leave the plan running as a savings vehicle and convert the whole loan to a capital and interest basis.

THE SEVEN AGES OF A GP
Registrar to 30 years old
- Secure membership of National Health Service Pension Scheme (NHSPS).
- Understand the core elements that make up the NHSPS.
- Take out building blocks of income protection, critical illness and life assurance.
- Mortgage commitments take priority.
- Do not over-commit. At this time other pension options can be delayed, if shortfall is not too great.

30 to 40 years old
- Retain membership of NHSPS.
- Take out locum insurance plan to protect against short-term disability.
- Look to tax efficient savings.
- Make a will.

40 to 50 years old
- Take out personal pension in respect of any non-NHS earnings, if appropriate.
- Consider added years (or AVCs) to top up shortfall in NHS service.
- Maintain insurance protection against death, sickness and retirement owing to ill health.
- Confirm with NHSPS office, Fleetwood, the current status of own pension benefits.

50 to 60 years old
- Consider maximising personal pensions on any non-NHS income or if you have short service.
- Maintain insurance protection against death, sickness and retirement owing to ill health.
- Start to plan towards retirement – again check pension benefits with Fleetwood.
- Review all savings and investments.

Retiring GPs
- Before retiring, obtain estimate of own pension and lump sum.
- Give notice required under partnership agreement.
- Give primary care organisation three months' notice.
- Make final contributions and review carefully.

- Explore open-market options and transfer all non-NHS pension funds if appropriate.
- Consider level pension as opposed to escalating payment for spouse, on AVC and personal pensions.
- Invest capital for a combination of growth and income.
- Address inheritance tax issues.

CHAPTER 12

Forward planning

This chapter can be broken down into the following five main sections.
- Why should we forward plan?
- Types and levels of forward planning.
- Preparing a detailed financial plan.
- Preparing a partner drawings forecast.
- Budgeting.

WHY SHOULD WE FORWARD PLAN?

> If you set off on a journey with nowhere in mind, then there is a good chance you will end up there. (Anon)

> There does in fact appear to be a plan. (Einstein)

> An intelligent plan is the first step to success. The man who plans knows where he is going, knows what progress he is making and has a pretty good idea when he will arrive. Planning is the open road to your destination. (Basil Walsh)

> You must have long-range goals to keep you from being frustrated by short-range failures. (Anon)

> It's not enough to be busy. The question is: what are we busy about? (Thoreau)

The finance partner's view
'With today's complexities in medical finance and pressure on practice income, our practice finds it essential to prepare financial forecasts for the year ahead. They provide the following benefits.
- Highlight the effect of major expenditure items such as partners' tax bills, superannuation shortfalls and partner maternity costs, together with the impact of major income items such as quality achievement pay.
- Allow partners to have a regular monthly income, helping with recruitment and retention.

- Give partners confidence that, given no major unforeseen events, the business finances are robust for the year ahead, thus allowing us to concentrate on getting our job done.
- Help prevent partnership arguments and disputes stemming from financial issues.'

Special reasons why a medical practice should plan ahead
- To foresee the effects of reduced levels of income.
- To ascertain the impact of a property move on the practice's normal finances.
- To plan a smooth transition for a practice merger or split.
- To give non-financial partners confidence to not worry about the practice's financial position.

TYPES AND LEVELS OF FORWARD PLANNING
Forward planning can encompass many things and may mean different things to different people. In a broader sense it could encompass strategic management, being the discipline of managing any organisation's resources to achieve long-term objectives. This can involve assessing the practice's current position, deciding where it wants to be in the future, and then assessing the actions needed to get it there. Tools such as SWOT analysis may be used whereby the practice's strengths, weaknesses, opportunities and threats are assessed, before arriving at a strategic plan developed to aid the practice in achieving its long-term objectives. These issues are outside the scope of this chapter where we are really concentrating on the subtopic of financial planning.

PREPARING A DETAILED FINANCIAL PLAN
Financial planning here relates to managing the financial resources of the practice, forecasting its future income and expenditure, budgeting for such and predicting how these affect the practice's cash flow.

Financial forecasting can be at varying levels. For example, a practice could prepare a daily or weekly cash flow prediction, or a monthly, quarterly or yearly forecast. We will look at a monthly financial forecast for the year ahead, later a monthly forecast for partners' drawings and finally budgeting.

Financial forecasts
Forecasting income
Take the latest available accounts and review each detailed line of income for anticipated changes in the year ahead. Identify items that will cease, start or change significantly. Assess correspondence from the primary care organisation as to the likely changes in your personal medical services budget or Minimum Practice Income Guarantee (MPIG). Assess what 'Enhanced Service' and

'Practice Based Commissioning' income may be available in the year ahead. Try to predict the timing of such. Allow for income from new services such as 'Extended Hours', and, of course, the costs of providing such services. Estimate changes in your quality income. For non-health authority income assume an inflationary increase of, say, 3%.

Table 12.1 shows an example of an income forecast prepared in March 2008.

Table 12.1 Example of income forecast prepared in March 2008

	2008–09 £
General medical services	
Global sum/MPIG (net of opt-out and employer's superann.)	571,200
PCO-administered income (seniority, maternity)	30,000
Enhanced services (various directed, national, local)	100,000
Quality and outcomes	228,000
Premises	140,000
	1,069,200
Other NHS income	22,500
Other non-NHS income	32,500
Reimbursement of expenses	118,000

A more detailed breakdown might look like Table 12.2.

Table 12.2 Example of income forecast prepared in March 2008 (detailed)

	2008–09 £
General medical services	
Global sum/MPIG (net of opt out and employer's superann.)	
Global sum	540,000
Less – opt out of services	(32,400)
Correction factor	150,000
Partners' employer's superannuation	(86,400)
Sub-total	571,200
PCO-administered income (seniority, maternity)	
Seniority	30,000
Enhanced services (various directed, national, local)	100,000

(continued)

	2008–09 £
Quality and outcomes	
Aspiration (70%)	156,000
Achievement	72,000
Sub-total	228,000
Premises	
Rent	100,000
Rates, water and refuse	40,000
Sub-total	140,000
	1,069,200
Other NHS income	
Dr X – Training grant	7,500
Dr Y – NHS Trust	7,000
Dr Z – PCT	8,000
	22,500
Other non-NHS income	
Companies	5,000
Insurance examinations, medicals and reports	25,000
Cremation fees	2,000
Donations received	500
	32,500
Reimbursement of expenses	
Registrars' salary and expenses	66,000
Staff training	2,000
Drugs	50,000
	118,000

Forecasting expenditure

Review each detailed line of expenditure incurred over the previous year and identify items that will change in the year ahead for known reasons. Otherwise, assume an inflationary increase of, say, 3%.

Table 12.3 shows an example of an expenditure forecast prepared in March 2008.

Table 12.3 Example of expenditure forecast prepared in March 2008

	2008–09 £
Expenditure	
Practice/medical expenses	83,200
Premises expenses	159,000
Staff expenses	377,710
Administration expenses	34,800
Finance expenses	11,000
	665,710
Other costs	
Depreciation	1,375
Interest expense/(income)	
Interest received	(1,254)

Table 12.4 shows a more detailed breakdown.

Table 12.4 Example of expenditure forecast prepared in March 2008 (detailed)

	2008–09 £
Expenditure	
Practice/medical expenses	
Drugs and consumables	45,000
Medical committee levy	4,200
Locum cover	9,000
Subscriptions including medical protection	25,000
Sub-total	83,200
Premises expenses	
Rent	100,000
Rates, water and clinical waste	40,000
Heat, light and power	6,000
Insurance (buildings)	2,000
Maintenance and repairs	3,000
Cleaning and laundry	8,000
Sub-total	159,000
Staff expenses	
Practice staff salaries and NIC	273,000
Staff pension costs	35,490

(*continued*)

	2008–09
	£
Registrars' salary and NIC and expenses	65,520
Staff training	2,500
Staff uniforms	1,200
Sub-total	377,710
Administration expenses	
Telephone	5,400
Postage, stationery and technical literature	7,200
Insurance (general)	1,200
Equipment repairs	1,000
Accountancy and legal charges	12,000
Sundry expenses	6,000
Advertising	2,000
Sub-total	34,800
Finance expenses	
Bank charges	1,000
Contingency	10,000
Sub-total	11,000
Other costs	
Depreciation	1,375
Interest expense	
Interest received	(1,254)

Other financial items to consider

As well as the obvious income and expenditure items, there are many other items of income and expenditure that need to be accounted for. What capital expenditure is anticipated, for example on equipment, furniture, property improvements, and so on? If the practice has loans or will need loans to finance capital items, bring the repayments into your forecasts. Is there a partner retiring in the year ahead? If so, you will have to provide for repayment of their capital or current account. Is there a partner joining and are they being asked to introduce capital into the practice? Partners' drawings are often left as the last item in your financial forecasts as they are likely to be paid from the surplus of income over expenditure (see below). Dispensing practices will need to consider the effect of VAT on their forecasts.

When considering these items, it must be appreciated that they do not affect the profitability of the practice as such, but they will have a significant effect on cash flow, which is dealt with later in the chapter.

An income and expenditure forecast for the year ahead

The above annual forecasts can be combined and broken down monthly to give a detailed annual forecast as shown in Table 12.5 on pp. 122–4.

Forecasting cash flow

While for simplicity we generally assume that income is earned and expenditure is incurred evenly across the year, money does not necessarily come and go from the bank account so evenly. A classic example of this is quality achievement pay. The full amount of quality income is earned across the year as GPs are working towards the quality measures. However, for 2008/09 the 'aspiration' portion (increased to 70%) is paid monthly throughout the year, with the balance of 'achievement' being paid typically in April, after the year end. Hence we can have income earned during the year but cash not received until the following year. All these timing differences have to be factored in to prepare a cash flow forecast. Typical items where cash flow timing differs from the earning of income or incurring of expenditure include the following:

- reimbursements – may be delayed
- insurance medicals – may be received one to three months in arrears
- seniority pay – earned evenly across the year but received quarterly
- partners' employer's superannuation – the shortfall or overpayment will be incurred during the year, but is likely to be balanced up by the PCO some 12 months after a March year end
- enhanced services – while the work may be carried out evenly across the year, the receipt of money for such may be sporadic
- rent expenditure to a third-party landlord – the expense is incurred evenly across the year, but payment is normally made quarterly
- rates – may be paid over 10 months or half-yearly or direct by the PCO
- insurance – may be paid once or by monthly instalments
- bank charges and interest – often occur quarterly
- drugs reimbursement – the receipt of cash-reimbursing drugs expenditure typically occurs two months late
- staff PAYE and pension deductions – typically there is a one-month delay before these deductions are paid over
- utility bills – this expenditure is incurred evenly across the year but may be paid quarterly, or by direct debit, with occasional balancing
- Medical Defence Union subscriptions
- partners' bonus drawings – this may occur as a one-off on top of regular monthly drawings
- partners' tax bills – if partners leave funds in the practice so that the practice can pay tax bills on their behalf, there will be large tax payments every six months, even though tax is being incurred evenly throughout the year in theory
- capital items – the purchase of a large piece of equipment may cause a one-off cash expense, but for accounting purposes the cost of the equipment may be spread over several years via depreciation.

Table 12.5 Doctor Example and Partners income and expenditure forecast for the year ending 31 March 2009

	Apr 08 £	May 08 £	Jun 08 £	Jul 08 £	Aug 08 £	Sep 08 £	Oct 08 £	Nov 08 £	Dec 08 £	Jan 09 £	Feb 09 £	Mar 09 £	Total £
General medical services													
Global sum/MPIG (net of opt-out and 'ers superan)	47,600	47,600	47,600	47,600	47,600	47,600	47,600	47,600	47,600	47,600	47,600	47,600	571,200
PCO-administered income (seniority, maternity)	2,500	2,500	2,500	2,500	2,500	2,500	2,500	2,500	2,500	2,500	2,500	2,500	30,000
Enhanced services (various directed, national, local)	8,333	8,334	8,333	8,333	8,334	8,333	8,333	8,334	8,333	8,333	8,334	8,333	100,000
Quality and outcomes	19,000	19,000	19,000	19,000	19,000	19,000	19,000	19,000	19,000	19,000	19,000	19,000	228,000
Premises	11,666	11,668	11,666	11,666	11,668	11,666	11,666	11,668	11,666	11,666	11,668	11,666	140,000
Total	89,099	89,102	89,099	89,099	89,102	89,099	89,099	89,102	89,099	89,099	89,102	89,099	1,069,200
Other NHS income													
Dr X – training grant	625	625	625	625	625	625	625	625	625	625	625	625	7,500
Dr Y – NHS Trust	583	584	583	583	584	583	583	584	583	583	584	583	7,000
Dr Z – PCT	667	666	667	667	666	667	667	666	667	667	666	667	8,000
Total	1,875	1,875	1,875	1,875	1,875	1,875	1,875	1,875	1,875	1,875	1,875	1,875	22,500

(continued)

	Apr 08 £	May 08 £	Jun 08 £	Jul 08 £	Aug 08 £	Sep 08 £	Oct 08 £	Nov 08 £	Dec 08 £	Jan 09 £	Feb 09 £	Mar 09 £	Total £
Other non-NHS income													
Companies	417	416	417	417	416	417	417	416	417	417	416	417	5,000
Insurance examinations, medicals and reports	2,083	2,084	2,083	2,083	2,084	2,083	2,083	2,084	2,083	2,083	2,084	2,083	25,000
Cremation fees	167	166	167	167	166	167	167	166	167	167	166	167	2,000
Donations received	–	–	–	–	–	–	500	–	–	–	–	–	500
Total	2,667	2,666	2,667	2,667	2,666	2,667	3,167	2,666	2,667	2,667	2,666	2,667	32,500
Reimbursement of expenses													
Registrars' salary and expenses	5,500	5,500	5,500	5,500	5,500	5,500	5,500	5,500	5,500	5,500	5,500	5,500	66,000
Staff training	167	166	167	167	166	167	167	166	167	167	166	167	2,000
Drugs	4,167	4,166	4,167	4,167	4,166	4,167	4,167	4,166	4,167	4,167	4,166	4,167	50,000
Total	9,834	9,832	9,834	9,834	9,832	9,834	9,834	9,832	9,834	9,834	9,832	9,834	118,000
Total income	103,475	103,475	103,475	103,475	103,475	103,475	103,975	103,475	103,475	103,475	103,475	103,475	1,242,200
Expenditure													
Practice/medical expenses	6,183	6,184	6,183	9,183	8,184	7,183	6,183	9,184	6,183	6,183	6,184	6,183	83,200
Premises expenses	13,250	13,250	13,250	13,250	13,250	13,250	13,250	13,250	13,250	13,250	13,250	13,250	159,000
Staff expenses	31,476	31,476	31,476	31,475	31,477	31,475	31,476	31,476	31,476	31,475	31,477	31,475	377,710
Administration expenses	2,900	2,900	2,900	2,900	2,900	2,900	2,900	2,900	2,900	2,900	2,900	2,900	34,800

	Apr 08 £	May 08 £	Jun 08 £	Jul 08 £	Aug 08 £	Sep 08 £	Oct 08 £	Nov 08 £	Dec 08 £	Jan 09 £	Feb 09 £	Mar 09 £	Total £
Finance expenses	916	918	916	916	918	916	916	918	916	916	918	916	11,000
Total	54,725	54,728	54,725	57,724	56,729	55,724	54,725	57,728	54,725	54,724	54,729	54,724	665,710
Other costs													
Depreciation	62	63	125	125	125	125	125	125	125	125	125	125	1,375
Interest expense/(income)													
Interest received	(131)	(232)	(244)	(135)	(39)	(65)	(89)	(108)	(113)	(55)	(14)	(29)	(1,254)
Excess income over expenditure	48,819	48,916	48,869	45,761	46,660	47,691	49,214	45,730	48,738	48,681	48,635	48,655	576,369
Cumulative excess	48,819	97,735	146,604	192,365	239,025	286,716	335,930	381,660	430,398	479,079	527,714	576,369	576,369

A cash flow forecast for the year ahead

If we take such differences into account we may arrive at a cash flow forecast for the year ahead as shown in Table 12.6 on pp. 126–8.

The predicted monthly bank balance shown at the bottom of the forecast may also be shown in graphical form as illustrated in Figure 12.1.

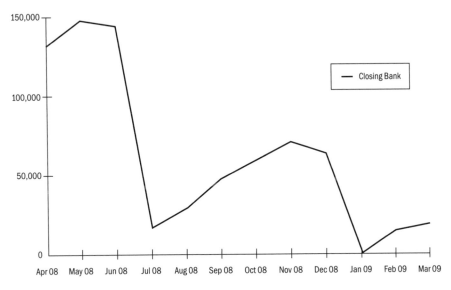

Figure 12.1 Predicted monthly bank balance.

Table 12.6 Doctor Example and Partners cash flow forecast for the year ending 31 March 2009

	Apr 08 £	May 08 £	Jun 08 £	Jul 08 £	Aug 08 £	Sep 08 £	Oct 08 £	Nov 08 £	Dec 08 £	Jan 09 £	Feb 09 £	Mar 09 £	Total £
Receipts													
Global Sum / MPIG (net of opt-out and 'ers superan)	51,800	46,800	46,800	46,800	46,800	46,800	46,800	46,800	46,800	46,800	46,800	46,800	566,600
PCO-administered income (seniority, maternity)	–	–	7,500	–	–	7,500	–	–	7,500	–	–	7,500	30,000
Enhanced services (various directed, national, local)	5,000	5,000	5,000	8,000	5,000	15,000	5,000	5,000	1,000	5,000	5,000	5,000	69,000
Quality and outcomes	101,143	11,143	11,143	11,143	11,143	22,285	13,000	13,000	13,000	13,000	13,000	13,000	246,000
Premises													
Rent	8,333	8,334	8,333	8,333	8,334	8,333	8,333	8,334	8,333	8,333	8,334	8,333	100,000
Rates, water and refuse	3,333	3,334	3,333	3,333	3,334	3,333	3,333	3,334	3,333	3,333	3,334	3,333	40,000
Sub-total	11,666	11,668	11,666	11,666	11,668	11,666	11,666	11,668	11,666	11,666	11,668	11,666	140,000
Dr X – Training grant	625	625	625	625	625	625	625	625	625	625	625	625	7,500
Dr Y – NHS Trust	583	584	583	583	584	583	583	584	583	583	584	583	7,000
Dr Z – PCT	667	666	667	667	666	667	667	666	667	667	666	667	8,000
Companies	500	500	417	416	417	417	416	417	417	416	417	417	5,167

(continued)

	Apr 08 £	May 08 £	Jun 08 £	Jul 08 £	Aug 08 £	Sep 08 £	Oct 08 £	Nov 08 £	Dec 08 £	Jan 09 £	Feb 09 £	Mar 09 £	Total £
Insurance examinations, medicals and reports	500	2,083	2,084	2,083	2,083	2,084	2,083	2,083	2,084	2,083	2,083	2,084	23,417
Cremation fees	167	166	167	167	166	167	167	166	167	167	166	167	2,000
Donations received	–	–	–	–	–	–	500	–	–	–	–	–	500
Registrars' salary and expenses	5,500	5,500	5,500	5,500	5,500	5,500	5,500	5,500	5,500	5,500	5,500	5,500	66,000
Staff training	167	166	167	167	166	167	167	166	167	167	166	167	2,000
Drugs	5,500	5,500	4,167	4,166	4,167	4,166	4,166	4,167	4,167	4,166	4,167	4,167	52,667
Interest received	–	–	–	607	–	–	239	–	–	310	–	–	1,156
	183,818	90,401	96,486	92,590	88,985	117,628	91,579	90,842	94,343	91,150	90,842	98,343	1,227,007
Payments													
Practice/medical expenses	10,933	6,184	6,183	9,183	8,184	7,183	6,183	9,184	6,183	6,183	6,184	6,183	87,950
Premises expenses	5,484	5,482	30,484	5,484	5,482	30,484	5,484	5,482	30,484	5,484	2,682	26,484	159,000
Staff expenses	24,408	24,867	24,865	25,466	24,866	24,865	24,865	24,867	25,465	24,866	24,866	24,866	299,133
Administration expenses	1,083	2,384	1,483	1,083	2,384	1,083	8,083	3,984	2,083	2,483	7,384	1,083	34,600
Finance expenses	833	834	1,083	833	834	833	833	834	1,083	833	834	1,083	11,000
Partners' drawings: Monthly	24,000	24,000	24,000	24,000	24,000	24,000	24,000	24,000	24,000	24,000	24,000	24,000	288,000

	Apr 08 £	May 08 £	Jun 08 £	Jul 08 £	Aug 08 £	Sep 08 £	Oct 08 £	Nov 08 £	Dec 08 £	Jan 09 £	Feb 09 £	Mar 09 £	Total £
Partners' drawings: Sundry – QOF/Equalisation bonus	–	–	–	48,000	–	–	–	–	–	–	–	–	48,000
Partners' drawings: Employees' superannuation	3,800	3,800	3,800	3,800	3,800	3,800	3,800	3,800	3,800	3,800	3,800	3,800	45,600
Partners' drawings – Added years	500	500	500	500	500	500	500	500	500	500	500	500	6,000
Partners' drawings: Taxation payments	–	–	–	90,000	–	–	–	–	–	80,000	–	–	170,000
Partners' drawings: NIC 2	92	92	92	92	92	92	92	92	92	92	92	92	1,104
Sub-total	28,392	28,392	28,392	166,392	28,392	28,392	28,392	28,392	28,392	108,392	28,392	28,392	558,704
Furniture, fixtures & fittings	–	–	–	5,000	–	–	–	–	–	–	–	–	5,000
PAYE/NI	6,000	6,510	6,510	6,510	6,510	6,510	6,510	6,510	6,510	6,510	6,510	6,510	77,610
Total payments	77,133	74,653	99,000	219,951	76,652	99,601	80,350	79,253	100,200	154,751	76,852	94,601	1,232,997
Net cash flow	106,685	15,748	(2,514)	(127,361)	12,333	18,027	11,229	11,589	(5,857)	(63,601)	13,990	3,742	(5,990)
Opening bank	25,000	131,685	147,433	144,919	17,558	29,891	47,918	59,147	70,736	64,879	1,278	15,268	25,000
Closing bank	131,685	147,433	144,919	17,558	29,891	47,918	59,147	70,736	64,879	1,278	15,268	19,010	19,010

Table 12.7 Doctor Example and Partners balance sheet forecast for the year ending 31 March 2009

	Opening £	Apr 08 £	May 08 £	Jun 08 £	Jul 08 £	Aug 08 £	Sep 08 £	Oct 08 £	Nov 08 £	Dec 08 £	Jan 09 £	Feb 09 £	Mar 09 £
Fixed assets													
Furniture, fixtures and fittings	15,000	15,000	15,000	20,000	20,000	20,000	20,000	20,000	20,000	20,000	20,000	20,000	20,000
Accumulated depreciation													
Furniture, fixtures and fittings	(10,000)	(10,062)	(10,125)	(10,250)	(10,375)	(10,500)	(10,625)	(10,750)	(10,875)	(11,000)	(11,125)	(11,250)	(11,375)
Sub-total	(10,000)	(10,062)	(10,125)	(10,250)	(10,375)	(10,500)	(10,625)	(10,750)	(10,875)	(11,000)	(11,125)	(11,250)	(11,375)
Total	5,000	4,938	4,875	9,750	9,625	9,500	9,375	9,250	9,125	9,000	8,875	8,750	8,625
Current assets													
Bank	25,000	131,685	147,433	144,919	17,558	29,891	47,918	59,147	70,736	64,879	1,278	15,268	19,010
Trade debtors	117,500	37,157	50,231	57,220	68,712	83,202	69,049	81,684	94,317	103,449	116,084	128,717	133,849
Other debtors	–	131	363	607	135	174	239	89	197	310	55	69	98
Stock of drugs	2,500	2,500	2,500	2,500	2,500	2,500	2,500	2,500	2,500	2,500	2,500	2,500	2,500
Total	145,000	171,473	200,527	205,246	88,905	115,767	119,706	143,420	167,750	171,138	119,917	146,554	155,457
Creditors due within one year													
Trade and other creditors	7,000	12,984	21,451	10,568	14,733	23,202	7,717	10,484	17,351	268	8,633	14,902	3,417
Net current assets	138,000	158,489	179,076	194,678	74,172	92,565	111,989	132,936	150,399	170,870	111,284	131,652	152,040
Total net assets	143,000	163,427	183,951	204,428	83,797	102,065	121,364	142,186	159,524	179,870	120,159	140,402	160,665
Capital and reserves													
Partners' current accounts b/fwd	63,000	63,000	63,000	63,000	63,000	63,000	63,000	63,000	63,000	63,000	63,000	63,000	63,000

	Opening £	Apr 08 £	May 08 £	Jun 08 £	Jul 08 £	Aug 08 £	Sep 08 £	Oct 08 £	Nov 08 £	Dec 08 £	Jan 09 £	Feb 09 £	Mar 09 £
Partners' drawings:													
Monthly	–	(28,300)	(56,600)	(84,900)	(113,200)	(141,500)	(169,800)	(198,100)	(226,400)	(254,700)	(283,000)	(311,300)	(339,600)
Sundry – QOF/ Equalisation bonus	–	–	–	–	(48,000)	(48,000)	(48,000)	(48,000)	(48,000)	(48,000)	(48,000)	(48,000)	(48,000)
Partners' drawings: Taxation provision	80,000	80,000	80,000	80,000	80,000	80,000	80,000	80,000	80,000	80,000	80,000	80,000	80,000
Partners' drawings: Taxation payments	–	–	–	–	(90,000)	(90,000)	(90,000)	(90,000)	(90,000)	(90,000)	(170,000)	(170,000)	(170,000)
Partners' drawings: NIC 2	–	(92)	(184)	(276)	(368)	(460)	(552)	(644)	(736)	(828)	(920)	(1,012)	(1,104)
Sub-total	80,000	114,608	86,216	57,824	(108,568)	(136,960)	(165,352)	(193,744)	(222,136)	(250,528)	(358,920)	(387,312)	(415,704)
Retained earnings	–	48,819	97,735	146,604	192,365	239,025	286,716	335,930	381,660	430,398	479,079	527,714	567,369
Total	143,000	163,427	183,951	204,428	83,797	102,065	121,364	142,186	159,524	179,870	120,159	140,402	160,665

Balance sheet forecast for the year ahead

A detailed understanding of a balance sheet may be beyond the readers' financial knowledge. Suffice to say that the balance sheet is the glue that holds the income and expenditure forecast and the cash flow forecast together, ensuring that the two reconcile with each other and confirming that no significant items have been forgotten about. A balance sheet forecast for the year ahead following on from the income and expenditure and cash flow forecasts shown in the two tables above might look like Table 12.7 on p. 129–30.

PARTNERS' DRAWINGS FORECASTS

1 As well as forecasting the overall practice finances, it is common to prepare a forecast of partners' monthly drawings for the year ahead. As we have seen, forecasting next year's income and expenditure often seems more of an art than a science, but the partners will want to know what their monthly drawings are likely to be. There are various methods used to calculate partners' drawings. These include: cash basis; accruals; two low months and higher for the quarter-end; evenly spread over 12 months; gross (with partners paying their own tax); and net (with the practice paying tax). Many practices with younger partners seem to appreciate evenly spread monthly drawings, as they find it helps to plan personal finances where sizeable personal mortgage payments and other commitments arise monthly.

2 Once the appropriate method is agreed, the next step is to project the practice's likely income and expenditure over the coming year. You may do this in great detail (as discussed above) if time allows, otherwise a rough estimate with a contingency may have to suffice.

3 The projected profit now needs to be divided among the partners. Are there likely to be any partner changes such as retirement, expansion, new partners or reduced commitments? Do prior shares of profit such as seniority or property profits need to be taken into account? What percentage will the balance of profit be shared in, and will this change during the year?

4 We now know our best guess at profit and how to share it out. Is that it? Unfortunately not, as we need to consider each partner's projected current account and the likely entries therein. Superannuation, including standard, added years, additional voluntary contributions (AVCs) and outside appointments will need reviewing. Tax, if paid by the practice, also needs to be looked at here. This can be complex and more so if the practice does not have a March year end. The balance needed on each partner's current account at the year end will need to be agreed, in line with the practice's working capital needs. There may be significantly lower needs if practices are PMS compared to GMS.

5 Now the easy bit – allow for a one-off QOF bonus, then the balance remaining on the current accounts can be divided by 12 to give the individual monthly drawings.

So what can we say to the manager or other individuals who have carried out this exercise? Congratulations, you've carried out the calculations, answered numerous queries, amended the spreadsheet countless times, told the partners that they can all have a drawings increase and everyone is happy. Before you go to sleep tonight perhaps just check that spreadsheet for any formula errors. Then of course there is the after-review. Following the next year end, review how actual figures compared to your projections. Explain to each partner why their actual current account differs from the projected version. If profits exceeded expectations, pay out 'bonus drawings'. If profits were lower, then hope that the contingency you allowed covers the shortfall. Good luck!

There are many ways of laying out such a forecast. One example of a partner drawings forecast is shown in Table 12.8, with the following assumptions:
- QOF achievement pay received in June 2009 is taken as bonus drawings
- seniority is included in the regular monthly drawings.

Table 12.8 Partners' drawings forecast

Anticipated profit available for distribution	£	£	£	£	£	£
Forecast excess of income over expenditure for the year						520,000
Less: Significant items affecting cash flow QOF achievement – not receivable until after year-end						–84,000
Contingency (already provided in forecast)						0
Balance available for distribution						436,000
Anticipated distribution of profit	Dr Prodit	Dr Pokit	Dr Treatit	Dr Curit	Dr Preventit	Total
Prior shares						
Seniority	9,328	5,942	3,296	653	620	19,839
Employer's superannuation	–13,000	–12,500	–14,500	–11,500	–11,500	–63,000
Balance distributed in profit sharing ratio	119,790	119,790	119,790	71,874	47,917	479,161
Total profit share	116,118	113,232	108,586	61,027	37,037	436,000
Anticipated profit sharing ratio %	25	25	25	15	10	100
Anticipated partner current accounts Balances brought forward 1 April 2009	15,500	16,500	16,000	10,000	7,000	65,000
Equalisation bonus to bring back into balance	–8,000	–9,000	–8,500	–5,500	–4,000	–35,000
Desired balances	7,500	7,500	7,500	4,500	3,000	30,000
Total profit share (as above)	116,118	113,232	108,586	61,027	37,036	436,000

(*continued*)

Anticipated profit available for distribution	£	£	£	£	£	£
Less: Various drawings						
Superannuation – standard	−6,967	−6,794	−6,515	−3,662	−2,222	−26,160
Superannuation – added years	−3,500	0	0	0	−1,200	−4,700
Tax and national insurance (paid by practice)	−40,000	−39,000	−36,000	−17,000	−7,000	−139,000
Less: Balance to carry forward	−7,500	−7,500	−7,500	−4,500	−3,000	−30,000
Balance to pay as monthly drawing	58,151	59,938	58,571	35,865	23,614	236,140
Monthly drawing	4,846	4,995	4,881	2,989	1,968	19,679

BUDGETING

Once a forecast for the year ahead has been made, the figures may also be used for budgeting purposes, and the monthly review of management accounts against those budgets. A sample budget is shown in Table 12.9.

Table 12.9 Practice management accounts for the six months ended 30 September 2009

	Month			Year to date			Full year
	Actual	*Budget*	*Variance*	*Actual*	*Budget*	*Variance*	*Budget*
Income	£	£	£	£	£	£	£
NHS income – GMS/PMS	77,000	79,167	−2,167	462,001	475,000	−12,999	950,000
Other NHS income	2,000	2,167	−167	15,002	13,000	2,002	26,000
Employer's superannuation	−4,000	−6,250	2,250	−24,000	−37,500	13,500	−75,000
Total NHS income	75,000	75,084	−84	453,003	450,500	2,503	901,000
Non-NHS income	1,000	2,500	−1,500	13,989	15,000	−1,011	30,000
Gross practice income	76,000	77,584	−1,584	466,992	465,500	1,492	931,000
Reimbursement of expenses	15,000	7,500	7,500	48,005	45,000	3,005	90,000
Total income	91,000	85,084	5,916	514,997	510,500	4,497	1,021,000
Expenditure							
Staff cost	25,405	25,000	−405	160,383	150,000	−10,383	300,000
Medical expenses	11,310	7,333	−3,977	48,740	44,000	−4,740	88,000
Premises	1,575	2,250	675	11,350	13,500	2,150	27,000

(*continued*)

	Month			Year to date			Full year
	Actual	*Budget*	*Variance*	*Actual*	*Budget*	*Variance*	*Budget*
Administration	4,240	2,000	−2,240	10,949	12,000	1,051	24,000
Finance	4,200	1,333	−2,867	7,845	8,000	155	16,000
Depreciation	0	300	300	0	1,800	1,800	3,600
	46,730	38,216	−8,514	239,267	229,300	−9,967	458,600
Bank interest received	0	83	−83	400	500	−100	1,000
Net practice income	44,270	46,951	−2,681	276,130	281,700	−5,570	563,400

Expenses may be broken down in detail for easier monitoring as shown in Table 12.10.

Table 12.10 Detailed breakdown of expenses

	Month			Year to date			Full year
	Actual	*Budget*	*Variance*	*Actual*	*Budget*	*Variance*	*Budget*
Staff costs	£	£	£	£	£	£	£
Practice staff	19,050	18,333	−717	121,000	110,000	−11,000	220,000
Staff pension	2,605	2,500	−105	15,025	15,000	−25	30,000
Staff training	0	83	83	300	500	200	1,000
Staff uniforms	0	84	84	0	500	500	1,000
Registrar's salary and expenses	3,750	4,000	250	24,058	24,000	−58	48,000
							300,000
Medical expenses							
Medical committee levy	200	208	8	1,301	1,250	−51	2,500
Deputising	2,500	1,375	−1,125	11,520	8,250	−3,270	16,500
Subscription including medical protection	1,600	1,667	67	9,902	10,000	98	20,000
Locum cover	4,000	750	−3,250	6,505	4,500	−2,005	9,000
Drugs	3,010	3,333	323	19,512	20,000	488	40,000
							88,000
Premises							
Rates, water and refuse	925	917	−8	5,600	5,500	−100	11,000
Heat and light	0	292	292	1,520	1,750	230	3,500
Insurance	0	208	208	0	1,250	1,250	2,500

(*continued*)

	Month			Year to date			Full year
	Actual	*Budget*	*Variance*	*Actual*	*Budget*	*Variance*	*Budget*
Maintenance and repairs	0	250	250	520	1,500	980	3,000
Cleaning and laundry	650	583	–67	3,710	3,500	–210	7,000
							27,000
Administration							
Telephone	2,010	458	–1,552	3,025	2,750	–275	5,500
Postage, stationery and technical literature	405	375	–30	2,906	2,250	–656	4,500
Equipment repairs	0	42	42	175	250	75	500
Computer expenses	1,500	167	–1,333	3,052	1,000	–2,052	2,000
Accountancy	0	542	542	0	3,250	3,250	6,500
Sundry expenses	325	250	–75	1,590	1,500	–90	3,000
Advertising	0	58	58	201	350	149	700
Legal and professional	0	8	8	0	50	50	100
Insurance	0	100	100	0	600	600	1,200
							24,000
Finance							
Bank charges	150	41	–109	295	250	–45	500
Property loan interest	4,050	1,292	–2,758	7,550	7,750	200	15,500
							16,000
Depreciation							
On fixtures, fitting and equipment	0	208	208	0	1,250	1,250	2,500
On computer	0	92	92	0	550	550	1,100
							3,600

CONCLUSION

If a practice is to take full control over the management of its finances, all of the above skills and practices are essential. However, a significant investment of time and money is normally required both to prepare and make regular use of such information. Modern, forward-thinking practices will consider such investments worthwhile and reap the benefits.

CHAPTER 13

The taxation of earnings

Since the advent of self-assessment, practice earnings are taxed on the individual. There is no longer a partnership liability to pay the income tax of the partners. However, some practices still save for their taxes within the partnership. This can be quite sensible if partners find it difficult to make the necessary savings. However, where partners have flexible mortgages, it can be cost-effective to use the tax savings to offset their mortgages, rather than leaving them in the practice to earn a comparatively low rate of interest.

Each partner or single-handed GP needs to complete a self-assessment tax return annually and submit it to HMRC. Tax returns (both partnership and personal) are issued in April each year and must now be filed by the following 31 October, for paper returns, or 31 January for online returns. Partners will need the partnership return completed first in order to complete their own personal partnership pages.

The partnership tax return is essentially derived from the accounts of the practice. The profit per the accounts should be adjusted for:
- items that are not tax deductible or taxable
- items that are taxable separately – such as taxed interest
- partners' expenses claims (if not included in the accounts)
- partners' capital allowance claims
- practice capital allowance claims.

This adjusted profit is then allocated between the partners in their profit-sharing ratios, taking account of items that are prior shared to individuals. Thus, for example, the taxable profits of the partners could be calculated as shown in Table 13.1. The partnership tax return includes details for each individual partner, which are then transferred to their personal tax returns.

Where a partnership return is late, there is an automatic penalty of £100 on the partnership *and* on each of the partners. This can be quite expensive in a large partnership.

The personal tax return will take the figures from the partnership return and

Table 13.1 Three-partner practice, accounts ending 31 March 2009

Profit per accounts			300,000	
Add back items that are not tax deductible				
Depreciation		2,000		
Employer's superannuation (if deducted in accounts)		25,000		
Life assurance		3,000		
			30,000	
			330,000	
Deduct items that are taxed separately				
Bank interest		200		
			200	
			329,800	
Deduct				
Practice capital allowances			3,000	
			326,800	
Partners' expenses claims				
Partner 1		1,200		
Partner 2		500		
Partner 3		1,500		
			3,200	
			323,600	
Partners' capital allowances				
Partner 1		1,000		
Partner 2		750		
Partner 3		1,200		
			2,950	
Taxable profits			320,650	
Allocate the profits:				
Profit-sharing ratios	*100*	*100*	*75*	*275*
	Partner 1	Partner 2	Partner 3	Total
Prior shares per accounts	12,000	8,000	3,000	23,000
Balance	108,236	108,236	81,178	297,650
Totals	120,236	116,236	84,178	320,650

include them on the partnership pages. It will also be necessary to show on the personal return any other income that is not already included in the partnership return. Great care must be taken by the GP or their accountant to ensure that the following pitfalls do not occur.

- It is easy to include income twice where it is retained personally but treated as part of the partnership accounts.
- Equally, it is easy to omit income that was thought to be part of the practice accounts, but was not.

To eliminate the risk of meeting these pitfalls it is probably best practice to include all medical income in the practice accounts and prior share anything that the partners agree is due personally.

HOW IS INCOME TAXED?

When the return is completed, the tax can be computed at the same time – or, if it is submitted prior to 31 October after the end of the tax year, the tax office will do the calculations. Normally, the accountant will carry out this work for GPs. All individuals are permitted to make some deductions from their total income before it is taxed, including:

- personal allowance
- superannuation contributions paid
- old-style retirement annuity premiums
- loan interest paid on a loan to buy a share of a partnership, or property used by a partnership.

Certain deductions attract relief only at higher rates (where the basic rate relief is obtained by paying net of tax in the first place), for example:

- gift aid payments to UK charities
- personal pension contributions.

After these deductions, tax is charged according to bands, which for 2008/09 are as follows:

- the first £36,000 at 20%
- the balance at 40%.

For those on very low incomes, there is a small 10% band for savings income, but this will not apply to practising GPs.

In addition to tax, Class 4 national insurance contributions must be paid, which are charged as follows:

- the first £5,435 is exempt
- the next £34,605 at 8%
- the balance at 1%.

Table 13.2 shows an example of a tax calculation for a typical GP.

Table 13.2 Personal tax computation for Doctor 1, tax year 2008–09

Share of partnership profit				120,236
Share of partnership interest				73
Personal interest				500
Total income				120,809
Deduct				
Superannuation contributions		25,000		
Interest on loan to buy into practice		1,500		
Personal allowance		6,035		
				32,535
Taxable				88,274
Tax on:				
First	34,800	20%	6,960	
Balance	53,474	40%	21,390	
				28,350
Class 4 NIC (on partnership profit, less practice interest paid)				
First	5,435	0%	–	
Next	34,605	8%	2,768	
Balance	78,696	1%	787	
				3,555
Total tax and NIC payable for the year				£31,905

WHEN IS THE TAX PAID?

For a continuing practice, the balance of tax is paid in the January following the end of the tax year (after payments already made on account), and a payment on account for the following year is made at the same time. Then, in July each year, there is a further payment on account. Using the example in Table 13.2, the tax-payment profile would be as shown in Table 13.3.

Table 13.3 Tax payment profile

Tax year 2008–09	£	£
Total tax calculated in Table 13.2		31,905
Payment dates		
31/01/2009 1st payment on account (based on 2007/08 tax) – say	10,000	
31/07/2009 2nd payment on account – as above	10,000	
		20,000

(continued)

Tax year 2008–09	£	£
31/01/2010 balancing payment		11,905
1st payment on account for 2009/10 (half of 08/09 tax)		15,953
Total due January 2010		27,858
31/07/2010 2nd payment on account (same as first)		15,953

WHAT HAPPENS IF RETURNS OR PAYMENTS ARE NOT MADE?

When a return is filed late, there is an automatic penalty of £100 and a further £100 if it is not filed by 31 July. If it continues to be unfiled, daily penalties of up to £60 per day can be imposed. Penalties can be remitted if it turns out that no tax is due – or restricted to the amount of tax due if it is less than the penalty (but note that penalties for late partnership returns are not restricted). Interest is automatically charged on late payment of tax with a 5% supplement if the January tax is not paid by the end of February and a further 5% surcharge if not paid by July. If returns are not made, there is a greater likelihood of an investigation into the individual's tax affairs by HMRC.

WHAT ELSE AFFECTS THE TAX CALCULATIONS?

Accounts that are made up to 31 March or 5 April are treated as being co-terminus with the tax year. If the accounts are made up to any other date in the year, it is the accounts date ending within the tax year that is used. For example, accounts made up to 30 June 2008 form the basis of the 2008–09 assessable profits. This can cause complications when a GP joins or leaves a practice, and a system of 'overlap relief' ensures that during the career of a GP all profits are taxed, and taxed only once.

Box 13.1 gives an example of a partner joining a practice.

Box 13.1

Using the profit shares from Table 13.1, but assuming accounts are made up to 30 June 2008, and that Partner 3 joined on 1 October 2007:

	Partner 1	Partner 2	Partner 3
Share of taxable profits	120,236	116,236	84,178

30 June 2008 falls in the tax year 2008/09 so these profits form the basis of the 2008/09 assessment for partners 1 and 2.

However, Partner 3 started on 1 October 2007 so these profits will be used for 2007/08 and 2008/09 for him or her.

2007/08 profits to be assessed will be those earned from start date to 5 April 2008 being 6 months of 9 months' earnings in the accounts to

30 June 2008.

Assessment for 2007/08 based on 6/9ths of 84,178 =   56,119*

2008/09   The accounts to 30 June 2008 do not include
          12 months' profits and so Partner 3 is assessed on:

          First 12 months in the practice:
          9 months to 30 June 2008 =   84,178
          3 months of accounts to 30 June 2009 say 25,000**
          Total   £112,178

* Note that these profits are taxed twice – once in 2007/08 and then again as part of
the 2008/09 assessment. This amount is carried forward as 'overlap relief'.

** This will be taxed again in 2009/10, so it will be added to the 'overlap relief' carried
forward.

The example in Box 13.2 shows how this overlap relief can be used when a GP
leaves the practice.

Box 13.2
Using the same figures in Table 13.1 but assuming that they relate to
accounts to 30 June 2008 and that Partner 1 retires on 30 June 2008:

For 2008/09 Partner 1 would be assessed on the profits arising in the
accounts for the year ended 30 June 2008   =   120,236

But this is 12 months' earnings and Partner 1 has only earned 3 months'
profits in the tax year. This would seem inequitable at first glance.

However, when Partner 1 first started in practice, he or she would have
been taxed twice on some of the profits – like Partner 3 in the example
above.

As profits will have increased over the years, the amount on which Partner
1 would have been taxed twice will be comparatively low.

If overlap relief had been, say,   25,000
Then this is deducted now to give assessable profits of   £95,236

Note:

These rules came into effect in 1996/97 and transitional overlap relief is available for those in practice at that time.

The effect of the rules is to ensure that practitioners are taxed once, and once only, on all the profits that they make during their time in practice.

WHAT FACTORS INFLUENCE THE CHOICE OF YEAR END?

A year end of 31 March is administratively simple to deal with as there are no complications or additional tax arising on leaving the practice. However, there is little opportunity to provide early warning of future taxation liabilities. Other year ends (particularly early in the tax year, such as 30 June) delay the payment of tax, which gives a cash flow advantage when profits are rising, but then gives rise to a higher tax liability in the year of cessation. However, tax can be calculated much earlier so that greater warning can be given of amounts of tax to be paid in the future. The comparison in Table 13.4 demonstrates the situation.

Table 13.4 Comparison of different year ends

Year ended 31 March		Tax year	Year ended 30 June	Profits pro-rate March figures	Reduction in taxable profits with June year end	If tax and NIC at 41%
2004	80,000	2003–04	2003			£ saving
2005	90,000	2004–05	2004	82,500	7,500	3,075
2006	110,000	2005–06	2005	95,000	15,000	6,150
2007	130,000	2006–07	2006	115,000	15,000	6,150
2008	130,000	2007–08	2007	130,000	–	–
2009	110,000	2008–09	2008	125,000	–15,000	–6,150

Thus it is clear that where profits are rising, tax is delayed when the accounts end early in the tax year, and these savings are significant where profits are rising quickly.

The converse would be true if profits were to fall.

Newly self-employed GPs must notify HMRC within three months of becoming self-employed, otherwise there is an automatic £100 penalty. Self-employed NIC (Class 2) must be paid, and these are normally paid by direct debit. The rate for 2008/09 is £2.30 per week. Incoming partners will experience a delay in paying tax but this eventually catches up with the GP and the first tax bill can come as a nasty shock. The example in Box 13.3 explains the situation.

Box 13.3 The timing of tax payments for a partner joining a practice
Using the details of Partner 3 in Box 13.1:

Profits assessable in 2007/08	56,119	
Profits assessable in 2008/09	112,178	

assume tax and NIC payable on these profits is

2007/08	12,000
2008/09	31,000

and that Partner 3 was previously employed, paying tax under PAYE and started with practice in October 2007.

Jan 08	no payment on account required, as no tax unpaid for 2006/07	–
Jul 08	no payment on account required, as no tax unpaid for 2006/07	–
Jan 09	tax for 2007/08 due	12,000
	plus payment on account for 2008/09	6,000
		18,000
Jul 09	payment on account for 2008/09	**6,000**
Jan 10	balance of 2008/09	19,000
	plus payment on account for 2009/10	15,500
		34,500
Jul 10	payment on account for 2009/10	**15,500**

LEAVING A PRACTICE

If a practice has a year end other than 31 March, the assessable profits in the last year may be higher than expected, as discussed earlier in the chapter. If a GP retires altogether or becomes employed, Class 2 NIC should be cancelled. If a GP is in receipt of a pension, in the year of retirement the tax code may well not deduct the correct amount of tax, and professional assistance should be sought to alleviate matters. If a GP leaves and joins another practice, it may become more complicated, with the need to use estimates at the initial stage. Professional assistance will inevitably be required, but the example in Box 13.4 provides at least a flavour of the calculations involved.

Box 13.4

Suppose that Partner 1 in Box 13.2 had left to join a new practice.

In 2008/09 he would have been assessed on income
relating to the old partnership profits, being: 95,236

If he then joined another practice with a September year
end:

then in 2008/09 for the new practice he or she would be
assessed on:

(assume profits of £130,000 pa in new practice)

1 July 2008 to 30 September 2008 say 32,500

6 months out of the accounts to 30 September 2009 say 65,000

(to 5 April 2009)

Total new practice 97,500

Total amount assessable in 2008/09 192,736

So while his or her practice income will have increased
only marginally (from 120,236 to 130,000)

his or her taxable income will have increased
from **120,236** to **192,736**

In practical terms GPs should note the following:
- September 2009 figures might not be available by January 2010.
- Tax due in January 2010 will include a payment on account for
  2009/10.
- 2009/10 will probably be lower than 2008/09 (perhaps based on
  profits of £130,000 + 5% increase – so £136,500) rather than the
  £192,736 calculated above.
- Thus it will probably be necessary to estimate the payments due –
  with the risk of an interest charge arising if the estimate is too low, or
  paying too much tax initially if the estimate is too high.

CHAPTER 14

Capital taxation

For many years capital transactions have been liable to taxation. Prior to 1965 there were limited ways in which capital was taxed, although we have had duty levied on assets held at death for over 100 years. This chapter is devoted to two forms of capital taxation:
- capital gains tax
- inheritance tax.

CAPITAL GAINS TAX

In line with income tax, capital gains are taxed by reference to the profit (or loss) arising in a year. The tax due is payable by 31 January following the tax year, i.e. for gains made in the year ended 5 April 2009, tax is payable by 31 January 2010.

Rates of tax

Up to 5 April 2008 the chargeable gain (gain less losses and after the annual exemption – see previous page) was considered to be additional income from savings. This was added to an individual's income from other sources and the extra tax payable at income tax rates is the capital gains tax (CGT) liability. From 6 April 2008, a flat rate of 18% applies to all gains, subject to reliefs.

Example
Dr Smith has a taxable income from other sources of £31,000 in 2007/08. He made a taxable gain on shares in that year of £6,000.

His CGT liability is calculated as follows:

		£
Balance of basic rate tax		
£34,600 – 31,000 =	3,600 @ 20% =	720

£2,400 @ 40% = 960

CGT payable by 31 January 2009 1680

Had the gain arisen in 2008/09, the CGT liability would be calculated as follows:

Taxable gain £6,000 @ 18% = £1,080 (payable 31 January 2010)

If personal allowances are unused, these cannot be offset against a capital gain.

Example

Mrs Smith, wife of Dr Smith, has no taxable income in 2008/09. She sells shares and a taxable gain of £8,000 arises.

Her CGT liability is calculated as follows: £8,000 @ 18% = £1,440

Mrs Smith's personal allowance of £5,435 is wasted.

Annual exemption

Each individual is entitled to tax-free capital gains of up to £9,600 for 2008/09 (£9,200 for 2007/08). Consequently, gains should be apportioned between husband and wife when possi ble to achieve the optimum saving of £19,200 tax-free gains.

Example

In 2008/09, gains are made by Dr Jones and his wife of £14,000 and £7,000 respectively. Upon the disposal of shares, the CGT liability would be:

	Dr Jones	Mrs Jones
Gains	£14,000	£7,000
Less annual exemption	9,600	7,000 (restricted)
Chargeable	4,400	Nil
Tax @ 18%	£792	£Nil

Had Dr Jones transferred some shares to his wife, who then subsequently sold them, the gains could be rearranged and equalised as follows:

	Dr Jones	Mrs Jones
Gains	£10,500	£10,500
Less annual exemption	9,600	9,600
Chargeable	900	900
Tax due	£162	£162

A saving of £468!

Losses

Losses will arise as well as gains. There is a pecking order for losses.
1 Losses must be offset against profits of the same year before the annual exemption.
2 Excess losses of a year can be carried forward and offset against future capital gains.
3 Losses brought forward are offset against gains which have been reduced by the annual exemption.

Spouses/civil partners

Married or registered couples are able to transfer or sell assets to each other without incurring a CGT liability. As mentioned above, this is useful where the annual exemption of a spouse has not been utilised, as a gain from the other spouse can effectively be transferred to make use of that exemption.

Who is liable?

An individual has to access their residence and domicile status. This is a complicated area and where doubt arises, professional advice should be sought.

Residence

In simple terms, an individual is resident in the UK if he or she has spent over six months in a tax year in the UK, or is in the UK on average for three months a year measured over a four-year period. For capital gains tax purposes, an individual is liable to CGT on gains if resident or ordinarily resident in the UK. Those who treat the UK as their home and live there normally are considered to be ordinarily resident and domiciled in the UK.

Domicile

This is a difficult concept to grasp. Domicile is considered to be the country an individual feels is his or her real home, i.e. somewhere he or she would normally live, but for circumstances that exist at that time. A person's domicile can be changed (domicile of choice). An individual not domiciled in the UK is not charged CGT on overseas assets unless the sale proceeds are brought into the UK.

Chargeable assets

Almost all types of assets are liable to CGT. It is easier to look at the exceptions. However, from a practical point of view GPs would normally come across only the sale of shares and property, as chargeable assets. The more common types of asset that are exempt from CGT are:
- one's own home (principal private residence)
- life assurance policies
- woodland

- gilt-edged securities, National Savings Certificates
- chattels, where sale proceeds do not exceed £6,000
- winnings and prizes from betting, premium bonds
- shares in an individual savings account (ISA) or personal equity plan (PEP)
- motor cars
- gifts to charities, etc.

How is capital gains tax calculated?

For most transactions the gain or loss is calculated by comparing the sale proceeds (or market value of a gift) with the cost of acquisition. Naturally, it is not quite as simple as that!

Sale proceeds

Generally, the proceeds of sale are used in the calculation. Expenses of the sale (e.g. estate agent and legal fees, stockbroker's commission) are deductible. There are exceptions to this rule when the sale is not at arm's length, i.e. where the sale is not at its true value. In these cases, market value is used instead. A typical example exists where an asset is sold to a family member at a favourable price. In this situation, market value is used. Similarly, when an asset is gifted, unless this is to a charity, the same rule applies.

What is the cost of acquisition?

In addition to the cost of the asset, the acquisition costs can be deducted in the CGT computation. These would include legal fees, surveyor's fees, advertising, stamp duties, etc. If an asset's value is enhanced, the costs of the enhancement can be claimed. From 2008/09, the base costs of assets held at 31 March 1982 is taken to be the market value at that date. Earlier costs are ignored.

Example

Dr Brown buys a house as a second home in 1974 for £300,000. He extends the premises in 1978 to provide a further bedroom, the cost of which is £70,000. The house is valued at 31 March 1982 at £480,000. The base costs for CGT is £480,000.

Other acquisition costs

Assets acquired from a deceased person's estate are transferred at probate value. Assets acquired from a spouse are transferred as original cost plus indexation (see below). Assets acquired as a gift are transferred at market value at the date of transfer.

Reliefs and allowances

In addition to the annual exemption, there have, over the years, been several reliefs and allowances, the more common of which are as follows.

Indexation

For the periods between 6 April 1965 and 30 April 1998, relief for inflation was given. The relief given was based on the increase in the retail price index between the month of acquisition and the month of disposal. Where the sale is after April 1998, the indexation relief is restricted. This relief is not available for disposal after April 2008.

Example

Dr White buys a chargeable asset in June 1989 for £25,000. He sells it in August 2008 for £150,000.

Dr White is not entitled to indexation allowance based on the increase in the retail price index between June 1989 and April 1998 (£10,225)

Sale price August 2008	£150,000
Cost June 1989	£25,000
Chargeable gain	£125,000

Taper relief

Indexation relief was replaced by taper relief after April 1998 but ceased for disposals after 5 April 2008. This relief was given by reference to the gain rather than the cost, and was calculated in accordance with the length of time the asset was held, and whether it was a business or non-business asset. This relief was calculated after indexation allowance and losses had been deducted.

The withdrawal of taper relief caused much upset, especially where business assets were concerned. Many business assets form part of an individual's retirement planning, and these assets were treated favourably by being taxed at an effective rate of 10%. Pressure on the government produced 'entrepreneur's relief' which applies to gains arising from 6 April 2008. This relief is a reduction of four-ninths of the chargeable business gain to produce an effective rate of 10% on the gross gain as prior to 5 April 2008.

Example

Dr White sells his share of his surgery premises in June 2008. A chargeable gain of £180,000 arises. Entrepreneur's relief of 4/9ths × £180,000 = £80,000 is given to reduce the gain to £100,000. Tax @ 18% is applied to this gain, i.e. £18,000. This is effectively a rate of 10% on £180,000.

The maximum amount on which relief can be claimed is £1 million. No such relief is available on non-business assets.

Main residence exemption

Any profit made on the sale of a main or only residence is exempt from capital gains tax. Various conditions must be satisfied. To be exempt from CGT, the property must be the only or main residence throughout the period of ownership. The exemption covers land and gardens of appropriate size, normally of up to 0.5 hectare. Where an individual is not resident in the property this technically makes the property liable to CGT for that period. However, there are several exceptions to that main rule and there are 'deemed' periods of residence whereby it is assumed the individual is resident, even if physically they are not. These deemed periods of residence include:

- period of up to 12 months between acquisition and the owner occupying the property
- the last 36 months of ownership, provided the property was at one time the individual's main residence
- periods of absence due to individual working abroad
- period of up to 48 months during which the owner returns to the property
- periods of up to 36 months provided the property is occupied both before and after as the individual's main residence.

If a home is let, the owner can claim lettings relief provided the property is let as residential accommodation. The relief is the lower of:
1 the main residence exemption
2 £40,000.

The relief is given to each owner of the property where jointly owned.

Example

Dr Field sold a freehold house in Southampton on 28 March 2009 for net proceeds of £252,220. She had bought the house for £15,000 on 1 October 1970 and immediately occupied it as her sole residence. Between 1 October 1972 and 1 April 1986 the house was let while she was employed in Suffolk, where she lived in rented accommodation. She resumed occupation of the house on 1 April 1986 but moved to a different permanent residence on 27 March 1988, the house then being let until the date of sale. The value of the house at 31 March 1982 was £70,000. To calculate the chargeable gain, the exempt proportion of the total period of occupation must be calculated.

Property was occupied from 31 March 1982 as follows:
31.03.82 to 31.03.86   4 years   Let while working away (resident before and after)

01.04.86 to 27.03.88	2 years	Owner-occupied
28.03.88 to 28.03.09	21 years	Let up to sale
	27 years	

The exempt proportion consists of actual and deemed periods of occupation:

Owner occupation	2 years
Allowable period of absence while working elsewhere in UK	4 years
Last 3 years	3 years
	9 years

	£
Sale proceeds March 2009	252,220
31 March 1982 value	70,000
Gain	182,220
Less exempt proportion 9/27	60,740
	121,480
Less residential lettings exemption	
Lower of £40,000 and exempt gain of £60,740	40,000
Chargeable gain	81,480

Property used for business or professional purposes may be liable to CGT. Where part of the home is used exclusively for the purpose of a trade or profession, that part does not attract main residence exemption. Doctors rarely use a room exclusively for practice purposes, although some GPs do use part of their home as their surgery. In this case, CGT will arise upon sale of the surgery part of the property. The average GP who uses a room as a study will normally use that room for other purposes, in which case a CGT liability will not arise.

Second home

Many GPs own second homes. An election can be made within two years of acquiring the second property to nominate one as the main residence. If this election is not made, the decision is made by HMRC based on fact. The second home would ordinarily attract a CGT charge upon sale.

Job-related accommodation

Job-related accommodation covers property that is provided to an individual to ensure the job is done properly, or for security purposes. In these circumstances, the individual can nominate a property owned as a main residence. The main residence exemption will therefore cover periods of non-residence even if let. This nomination can be made by either employed or self-employed individuals.

Quoted stocks and shares

The rules relating to quoted securities are complex, especially with regard to the identification of shares where only part of a holdings is sold.

A brief summary of the basic rules of identification will assist those who have simple calculations.

Where shares are sold, they are matched:

- with acquisitions on the same day
- with acquisitions made within 30 days
- with acquisitions being treated as having come out of a pool. All acquisitions of shares of the same class are treated as forming a single pool, with shares coming out at average costs.

Chattels

Assets that are not shares or property, but are tangible, such as furniture, pictures, and the like, are liable for CGT where the sale proceeds exceed £6,000. The chargeable gain is then restricted to five-thirds of the excess over £6,000.

> **Example**
> An antique clock is sold for £7,800. The clock was purchased for £3,000. The chargeable gain is restricted to $5/3 \times 1,800$, i.e. £3,000.

Capital gains tax planning

Capital gains are taxed in the year of disposal at the marginal (highest) rate of income tax. The gain will in many cases be an accumulation of gains over several years, resulting in a high tax charge. To mitigate or cancel a tax charge often requires professional advice, but there are ways to reduce a CGT charge. The use of both spouses' annual exemptions is a simple way of optimising this relief. Transfers of assets between husband and wife are not subject to tax and consequently the transfer of a gain from one spouse to another to utilise the annual exemption makes sense. Furthermore, one can use the tax-free transfer method to transfer assets from one spouse to the other where the recipient spouse has capital losses from an earlier year.

> **Example**
> Dr Grey is to sell an asset that will make a gain in 2008/09 of £30,000. Mrs Grey has capital losses of £10,000 brought forward from a previous year. To utilise the losses, the asset should first be transferred by Dr Grey to his wife who will then sell it to produce a gain of £30,000.
>
> Mrs Grey's position will be:
> Gain   30,000

Less losses	10,000
	20,000
Less exemption	9,600
Chargeable gain	£10,400

Up to 2007/08, a transfer of assets between spouses was also a useful way of taxing a gain at the lower rate of tax, but is now no longer available.

As the annual exemption of £9,600 cannot be carried forward where not utilised, if a gain can be created and the asset bought back, the base cost of the asset can be increased by up to the value of the annual exemption.

Example
Dr Silver sells shares to produce a capital gain of £8,000. This is covered by the annual exemption and no tax is payable. Mrs Silver buys shares at the higher value. A future profit will be reduced by the increased cost and will attract a further annual exemption when sold, thereby releasing tax-free gains of up to £19,200 (2 × £9,600).

INHERITANCE TAX
Introduced over 20 years ago, this tax is generally payable on death, although there are situations where a charge can be created on lifetime gifts. As these occasions are restricted, no further reference will be made to them.

An individual who is domiciled in the UK is liable to inheritance tax (IHT) on worldwide assets. A non-UK domiciled individual is liable to IHT on UK assets only.

IHT at 40% is payable on all chargeable transfers (gifts) in excess of the exempt band of £312,000 for 2008/09. The exempt band is increased to £325,000 for 2009/10.

Example
Dr Silver dies and his estate is valued at £717,000 with debts outstanding of £5,000. The IHT payable is:

Value of estate	717,000
Less debts	5,000
	712,000
Exempt	312,000
Chargeable @ 40%	£400,000

IHT of £160,000 is payable.

Gifts made in one's lifetime are liable to IHT if death occurs within seven years of making that gift. These gifts are called potentially exempt transfer (PETs). Where the donor survives seven years the gift is exempt only if made to an individual or to certain types of trust. A record of gifts should be maintained by all donors. If the gift is not exempt, the value of that gift is added to the deceased's estate for IHT calculation purposes. There is taper relief when gifts are made between three and seven years before death, which reduces the tax payable.

Exempt gifts or transfers

Certain gifts will not attract IHT:
- gifts to a spouse or civil partner
- individual gifts of up to £250 in any one tax year. There is no limit to the number made
- £3,000 annual exemption. This covers the whole part of a gift not otherwise exempt. Any unused part of this exemption can be carried forward one year only
- gifts to charities of any amount
- gifts to certain museums, art galleries, National Trust for the benefit of the nation
- gifts in consideration of marriage to bride or groom. The exempt amount depends on the status of the donor:
  - each parent can give up to £5,000
  - each grandparent or great-grandparent can give up to £2,500
  - the bride or groom can give up to £2,500
  - any other person can give up to £1,000
  - gifts out of income can be treated as normal expenditure and exempt from tax. Typical examples include life assurance premiums, and regular payments to support a relative where the gifts do not affect the donor's normal standard of living.

Business property and agricultural reliefs

Provided the property has been owned for two years, relief of up to 100% is given at death. If the property is owned by a sole proprietor or single-handed GP, 100% relief is given. If the property owned is used in a partnership, 50% relief is given.

Example

Dr Grey dies. Among his estate is a part share in the surgery premises valued at £60,000. Business relief of £30,000 is to be added into his estate. Agricultural relief at 100% is available in certain situations where the individual has occupied the farmland. This is a specialist area and professional advice should be sought.

IHT planning

To plan for one's death is difficult for many, but GPs are human and inevitably death will occur. The main problem is when it occurs. Plans can be made, but it is the timing of events that often upsets these. Regular reviews are therefore necessary. The first step is for the GP to ensure that he or she has an up-to-date will. Do not ignore the making of a will, as the intestacy rules which will apply are complex, expensive and unlikely to achieve your wishes. If married, this applies to the spouse also. The will contains instructions which will be put into operation upon demise and will cover not only the financial arrangements, but also the question of guardianship and trusteeship for minor children.

The will can be drawn up to contain a discretionary will trust. This allocates the exempt part of the estate on death (£312,000) to a trust operated by the trustees at their discretion, where ordinarily a person might leave the whole of their estate to their spouse or civil partner. As mentioned above, transfers to a spouse or civil partner are exempt and until 8 October 2007 the exemption of £312,000 would be lost. This trust arrangement potentially saved £124,800 inheritance tax (at 40%).

For deaths after 8 October 2007, the unused nil-rate band of a spouse can be claimed by the survivor upon his or her death. The relief is based on any unused nil-rate band available from 26 March 1974 (when IHT was introduced), but revalued to the nil-rate band at death.

Example

Mrs White died in December 2005. Her nil-rate band of £275,000 was unused as all assets were transferred to her husband.

Dr White died in March 2008. His executor will be able to claim £300,000 relief brought forward (the nil-rate band for 2007/08 together with the nil-rate band of £300,000) for Dr White. The total relief is therefore £600,000.

The creator of a discretionary live trust will in many cases be considered now to be obsolete. However, professional advice should be taken before making any decisions as trusts do have other benefits, such as the reduction of assets where funding for long-term care is required.

Savings at death are restricted, e.g. gifts to charities, and planning with action before death is necessary to make savings to allow more of one's estate to be gifted to children and others. Savings can possibly be made at death through a deed of variation, which allows beneficiaries to change the contents of a will. Professional advice must be sought in these circumstances. Lifetime action usually requires the donor to survive seven years. This must be borne in mind to achieve optimum savings.

Equalisation of estates of married couples is recommended, not only for IHT purposes, but also for income tax. Each individual should have assets, where possible, equal to at least the exemption at death (£312,000).

The use of exemptions and reliefs is important, provided that the gift can be afforded. Those with excess assets that they wish to transfer to children, grandchildren, etc., should consider affordable transfers beyond the exemptions. If the seven-year period is survived, the gifts become exempt. Leaving the gift until later in life shortens the odds.

The use of life assurance policies is attractive to some individuals. These policies are put into trust outside an individual's estate to escape IHT. The funds can be used to make gifts to beneficiaries and/or provide funding to pay IHT. Advice from an independent financial advisor is necessary.

Bearing in mind a gift of £1,000 can save IHT of £400, it makes sense to discuss and plan. Your accountant knows you and your circumstances well – the earlier these issues are dealt with the better.

CHAPTER 15

VAT and the GP

GENERAL

Prior to 1993, general practitioners were blissfully ignorant of the delights of VAT; however, since HMRC recognised them as independent contractors that has changed. This has resulted in GPs asking their advisors, 'Should I be registered for VAT?' The pleasures of VAT are such that although the basic question remains 'Should I be registered', the factors to be considered have changed since 1993.

So before looking at current considerations let's revisit some of the key events and dates to try and make sense of the present situation.

KEY DATES

1972

VAT was introduced and HMRC took the view that GPs were part of the NHS and not independent contractors. They were therefore not considered to be in business, income was deemed to be outside the scope of VAT and they could not register for VAT.

1993

HMRC Press Release 44/93 confirmed that GPs were now to be treated as independent contractors; the supply of medical services therefore became exempt rather than outside the scope of VAT. This paved the way for the short-lived 'Toothbrush Scheme' registration where, by making negligible standard-rated sales such as 'travel packs', practices were able to register voluntarily for VAT and reclaim up to £7,200 VAT on overheads due to the partial exemption *de minimis* rules in existence at that time. Needless to say, HMRC was not going to let that situation continue for long!

30 November 1994

Changes in the partial exemption *de minimis* rules meant the end for Toothbrush Schemes. Prior to that date, if the practice was partially exempt but exempt input tax was less than £600 per month on average, it could all be recovered. Subsequently, although the monthly amount was raised to £625, exempt input tax had not to exceed 50% of the total input tax for the period. Interestingly, the amount of £625 has remained unchanged since 1994.

1995

HMRC recognised that the supply of drugs by a GP providing NHS pharmacy services could be zero rated, giving dispensing practices the opportunity to register and reclaim a proportion of their overheads under the partial-exemption rules. The level of their zero-rated inputs meant they did not fall foul of the 50% *de minimis* rule introduced in November 1994.

2002

The Court of Appeal decision in the Benyon case reversed the earlier High Court finding and held that drugs personally administered by a GP were to be treated as zero rated rather than part of an exempt medical service. This significantly increased the repayment of VAT received by VAT-registered practices.

2003

The European Court of Justice issued its judgement in the case of Dr d'Ambrumenil. The decision of the Court affected the way in which the UK viewed the VAT exemption for health and as a result of this the VAT treatment of some services changed and this led to some practices being required to register for VAT.

2004

The House of Lords reversed the Court of Appeal decision in the Benyon case and personally administered drugs are once again exempt. The significant increase in VAT repayments received after the Court of Appeal decision not only stopped but actually had to be repaid to HMRC. The Statement of Financial Entitlements states that the reimbursement for drugs from the Prescription Pricing Authority will include an allowance for VAT based on the pre-discount value.

The combined impact of these two events created serious doubts as to whether it remained financially advantageous for GPs to be registered for VAT.

2005

Meetings between the GPC and Department of Health confirmed that the change in the method of calculation of VAT allowance between the Statement of Fees and Allowances (SFA) and the SFE was a mistake by the drafters. It was never intended that VAT would be reimbursed based on a pre-discount value and a retrospective change to the SFE was agreed and VAT is now reimbursed on the cost net of discount. So once again there was yet another about-turn in circumstances that practices and their advisors needed to review when considering registration.

2006

The General Medical Services Contract Review Negotiations 2005/06 resulted in two significant changes:
1 from 1 April 2006, the DoH will pay a VAT allowance on personally administered drugs, and
2 from 1 April 2006, no VAT allowance will be paid by the PPA on items dispensed by GPs.

This forces dispensing practices to register for VAT as the only means of reclaiming the VAT incurred on the purchase of drugs prescribed to dispensing patients.

On 15 December 2006, HMRC issued *VAT Information Sheet 12/2006 – Further information for dispensing doctors*. This sheet provided further guidance on some of the queries that had arisen in practice in the period since 1 April 2006 when most dispensing practices registered.

2007

On 30 January 2007, HMRC issued *Revenue & Customs Brief 06/2007 VAT – Changes to the exemption for medical services*. This document gave advance notice of HMRC's decision to implement the Dr d'Ambrumenil decision from 1 May 2007.

KEY CASES

The key dates above highlight two cases which have had a significant influence on the past and present scenario of GPs and VAT, and accordingly further details are given below.

Benyon case

The practice supplied drugs and appliances personally to patients in rural areas under Regulation 20 of the National Health Service (Pharmaceutical) Regulations 1992. It was accepted that the prescription of drugs under such circumstances was zero rated within Schedule 8, Group 12, Item 1A, VAT Act 1994. The issue was whether drugs and appliances personally administered or applied to the patient by the practice were also zero rated.

In the earlier case of Dr Woodings, Rees, Crossthwaite and Jones, the VAT Tribunal had found that the supply of the goods was dissociable from the exempt supply of medical care. However, in the Benyon case the Tribunal held that there was a single composite exempt supply of medical care and dismissed the appeal.

This was the start of a roller-coaster ride which found the High Court confirming that a single supply exempt medical service was made. This decision was then reversed by the Court of Appeal before being confirmed in the final twist by the House of Lords.

Dr d'Ambrumenil

The case of Peter d'Ambrumenil, Dispute Resolution Services Ltd v Commissioners of Customs & Excise was referred to the Court by the VAT and Duties Tribunal, London on the interpretation of Article 13A(1)(c) of Sixth Council Directive 77/388/FEC of 17 May 1977.

The case centred on the tax treatment of certain activities of the appellants. The activities involved acting as an expert witness in medical negligence, personal injury and disciplinary proceedings; and arbitration and mediation services which required both legal and medical expertise.

The Commissioners of Customs & Excise concluded that several of these activities fell within the scope of Item 1 in Group 7 in Schedule 9 to the VAT Act 1994 and were therefore exempt from VAT. Dr d'Ambrumenil appealed against this decision and the VAT and Duties Tribunal decided to stay proceedings and refer to the Court.

The decision of the Court on 20 November 2003 was that the exemption from VAT applies to medical services consisting of:
- conducting medical examinations for employers or insurance companies
- the taking of blood or other bodily samples to test for the presence of viruses, infections or other diseases on behalf of employers or insurers, or
- certification of medical fitness, for example as to fitness to travel where for example those services are intended principally to protect the health of the person concerned.

The said exemption does not apply to the following services performed in the exercise of the medical profession:
- giving certificates as to a person's medical condition for purposes such as entitlement to a war pension
- medical examinations conducted with a view to the preparation of an expert medical report regarding issues of liability and the quantification of damages for individuals contemplating personal-injury litigation
- the preparation of medical reports following examinations referred to in the previous point and medical reports based on medical notes without conducting a medical examination
- medical examinations conducted with a view to the preparation of expert medical reports regarding professional medical negligence for individuals contemplating litigation.

HMRC chose to implement this decision with effect from 1 May 2007. As a result of this decision it is possible that some practices may need to register for VAT, but more importantly practices that are already registered must remember to account for VAT on any outputs caught by the new rules.

REGISTRATION

Despite the succession of changes since 1993, the fundamental question aimed at advisers is still: 'Should a practice be registered?' The answer is still based on three considerations.

- Does the practice have a legal requirement to register?
- If there is no legal requirement, is it possible to apply for voluntary registration?
- If voluntary registration is possible, is it in the practice's interest to do so?

Unfortunately, these simple questions have been complicated by the various changes detailed above, not to mention the fact that many practices do not wish to incur the additional administrative burden of registering for VAT.

Does the practice have a legal requirement to register?

For registration to be required a practice must make taxable supplies over the current registration threshold of £67,000. Most practices only believe they make exempt supplies through their medical services; however, dispensing practices make zero-rated supplies where they are required to provide NHS pharmacy services to their patients. In many cases these taxable supplies will put them over the VAT registration threshold.

Prior to 1 April 2006, even where the level of zero-rated sales was over the threshold it was possible to elect not to register for VAT and reclaim the VAT via the PPA. However, from that date the PPA will no longer refund VAT to GPs on items dispensed over the counter, in effect forcing GPs to register for VAT.

In addition, the decision in the Dr d'Ambrumenil case means that practices may have additional income which is now categorised as a taxable supply and means the registration threshold is reached.

Is it possible to apply for voluntary registration?

If a practice makes zero or standard-rated supplies, but at a level below which there is no legal requirement to register, they may still apply for voluntary registration. This leaves the following key questions.

- Is the practice financially better off by registering?
- Is the financial gain worth the additional administrative burden?

Financial implications

The recent changes whereby the PPA will not refund VAT on drugs dispensed over the counter has led to a clear distinction between dispensing and non-dispensing practices with taxable supplies below the registration level.

Dispensing practices

The potential loss of the 17.5% VAT on drug costs alone could be sufficient to justify registration. Drugs with a cost of £40,000 could potentially result in the loss of £7,000 VAT refund. In addition, a proportion of overheads could be recovered in the partial exemption rules but beware some VAT may need paying on activities which are now classed as taxable following on from the Dr d'Ambrumenil decision.

Non-dispensing practices

It is hard to see any situation where voluntary registration would be worthwhile. VAT would have to be accounted for on services now taxable following the d'Ambrumenil decision. It is unlikely there would be significant input VAT to recover on these taxable activities and the proportion of input VAT recoverable through the partial exemption calculation is likely to be minimal.

In summary, the costs in time and effort are almost certain to outweigh the potential VAT recovery.

VAT REGISTRATION – THE ISSUES

Once the question of registration has been determined, the practice is faced with completing a VAT return on a monthly or quarterly basis in accordance with the partial exemption rules. While not wanting to go through in detail those rules which can be found in standard VAT texts, it is worthwhile looking at the factors which you would expect to appear in a practice's VAT calculation.

Calculation of VAT recovery

The calculation of the VAT recovery has been split into three steps:

Outputs
- Analysing the outputs to determine output tax payable and the percentage of non-attributable input tax.

Inputs
- Analysing inputs to determine how much is recoverable in full as it relates to taxable supplies.
- Determining that which is wholly irrecoverable as it relates to exempt outputs.
- Determining that which is not attributable wholly to either of the former and which is therefore recovered in accordance with the rate calculated above for non-attributable input tax.

Net amount recoverable
- The calculation of net amount recoverable based on the stages detailed above.

An illustration of how this works is given in Table 15.1.

Table 15.1 Example of VAT recovery calculations
VAT outputs

	Notes	Total Ex-VAT	Exempt	Taxable	VAT
		£	£	£	£
GMS2	1	1,150,000	1,050,000	100,000	
Other income					
Medical services		20,000	20,000		
Other income					
Non-medical services	2	30,000		30,000	5,250
Dispensing					
To dispensing patients		220,000		220,000	
Personally administered	3	40,000	40,000		
		1,460,000	1,110,000	350,000	5,250

Taxable % = 350,000/1,460,000 = 24% (Note 4)

Allocation of input VAT

	Total Ex-VAT	VAT	Exempt	Taxable	Non-attributable
	£	£	£	£	£
Expenditure					
Staff expenses	200,000	–			
Premises	25,000	500			500
Practice expenses					
Other	45,000	–			
Other (Non-medical services)	1,000	175		175	
Drug purchases	200,000	35,000		35,000	
Self-administered drug purchases	40,000	7,000	7,000		
Administrative expenses	75,000	8,000			8,000
Finance expenses	1,000	–			
	587,000	50,675	7,000	35,175	8,500

VAT recovery

VAT output tax	(5,250)
VAT input directly attributable	35,175
Proportion of input tax on	
Non-attributable VAT £8,500 × 24% (Note 8)	2,040
Total VAT recoverable	31,965

The basic calculations shown in Table 15.1 are quite straightforward, but as usual the devil is in the detail and listed below are some of the areas which will need special attention.

Notes
1 Some income sources received under the GMS or PMS contract are consideration for both taxable (in this case zero-rated) and exempt supplies. For example, GMS global sum, MPIG correction factor, notional rent.
2 Following the d'Ambrumenil decision, it will be necessary to review all non-GMS sources of income to determine the VAT treatment. The essential point here is *all* income, not just the certificates, but any contracts with business or educational establishments for example. Remember, in accordance with the events discussed under 'Key dates' at the start of the chapter, it is the purpose of the activity that is essential.

   Having identified these items, it is necessary to have an accounting system which will record them and assist with the preparation of the VAT return, in particular accounting for the VAT that is due on their outputs.
3 In accordance with the decision in the Benyon case, personally administered drugs are exempt and therefore need to be separated and recorded as such on the accounting system. HMRC will accept that a reasonable method of calculating the reimbursement relating to personally administered drugs is to take the VAT allowance received on the drug statement from the PPSA and multiply this by 100%/17.5%.
4 In a partially exempt situation, only a proportion of the VAT on inputs which are not directly attributable to exempt or taxable supplies can be reclaimed. This proportion is usually calculated on the standard method, i.e. the proportion of taxable income (including zero rated) to total income. In this example, arriving at a rate of 24%. However, it should be remembered that other methods can be used to calculate the proportion of non-attributable VAT recoverable, perhaps floor space, but any such method will need agreeing with HMRC.
5 When allocating input VAT, it is important to remember that any that relates directly to other income taxable following the d'Ambrumenil decision needs identifying as it will be recoverable in full.
6 Following the Benyon decision, the VAT on personally administered drugs has to be identified and recorded as this is exempt and not recoverable.
7 Any expenses which are not attributable directly to exempt or taxable activities go into the non-attributable column and a percentage is recoverable in accordance with Note 3 above.
8 The calculation for the non-attributable tax recoverable has to be done separately each quarter. However, an annual adjustment takes place each year when a percentage calculated over the year is applied to adjust for any inequities which may have occurred quarter by quarter.

It is also worth remembering the *de minimis* rules, such that if exempt input tax is less than £625 per month (the total input tax directly attributable to exempt outputs and the amount of the exempt proportion of non-attributable input VAT) and exempt input tax has not exceeded 50% of the total input tax, all the exempt VAT is recoverable.

PREMISES DEVELOPMENTS

Prior to the proposed changes from 1 April 2006, dispensing practices sometimes registered for VAT to reclaim input VAT on a major property development. The new circumstances mean that those practices will probably already be registered and so this will no longer be a major planning consideration. However, there may be possibilities for non-dispensing premises to register based on earnings that are taxable under the d'Ambrumenil ruling.

This is a situation which requires careful consideration with advisers, particularly as the Capital Goods Scheme (land, buildings, civil engineering works and refurbishments with a VAT exclusive value of £250,000 or more) may be involved and the practice may be locked into registration for a number of years, which may dilute the advantage gained. More details on the Capital Goods Scheme can be obtained from C&E Notice *706/2*.

HMRC GUIDANCE

Because of the piecemeal manner in which VAT as it affects doctors has developed, one has to refer to a number of different documents to build up the full picture of HMRC's views. At the time of writing guidance can be found in the following documents.

- VAT Information Sheets:
  - 03/06 (January 2006) *Dispensing doctors and VAT registration*
  - 12/06 (December 2006) *Further information for dispensing doctors*
  - 05/07 (February 2007) *Health professionals affected by changes to exemption for medical services*
- VAT Notice
  - 701/57 (January 2007 edition) *Health professionals*
  - HMRC VAT Manual
  - VATHLT 2010–2150

THE FINAL WORD

The difficulties created for practices in dealing with VAT are well illustrated with the uncertainties over the VAT treatment of fees received for issuing cremation certificates. The VAT manual states that such fees were exempt from VAT before 1 May 2007 but that from 1 May 2007 they would be standard rated. Presumably, this was on the basis that the principal purpose of the service couldn't be the protection, maintenance or restoration of the health of an individual, given that the individual in question had already died! However, a Written Enquiries Officer had advised an AIMSA member that fees payable for certified copies of cremation certificates were completely outside the scope of VAT as they were paid in fulfilment of a statutory requirement. There was then further argument that fees for 'Form B' certificates, which can only be issued by the doctor who attended the deceased before their death, would be outside the scope of VAT, but fees for 'Form C' certificates, which can be issued by any doctor with the appropriate experience, would be standard rated. After some weeks of confusion the final answer was that all such fees would remain exempt, but not because of the rules that apply to doctors, but under a completely different section of the VAT legislation that relates to undertakers. Notwithstanding this 'final' decision, the VAT manual published by HMRC for use by VAT officers still states that fees for cremation certificates are standard rated!

All this goes to show that the medical profession will continue to require a good deal of assistance and education if it is to keep up with all the changes and this will undoubtedly provide opportunities for the proactive advisor.

CHAPTER 16

A compilation of financial tit-bits

The contributors to this book are all members of the Association of Independent Specialist Medical Accountants, which publishes a quarterly newsletter on current financial issues affecting medical practice. We now select a number of articles that have stood the test of time and remain of interest to GPs. The articles selected and reproduced below are as follows.

- Inheritance tax – relevant but overlooked
- GP-owned pharmacies – an opportunity?
- Staff pay – dictated by business decisions?
- Surgery premises – an interesting tale
- Where is the goodwill?
- From manager to partner
- Another tax time bomb waiting to explode
- Capital accounts made easy
- Stamp duty land tax and medical partnerships
- Buying in to a practice
- Equalisation of partnership shares
- Practice-based commissioning – an overview
- Partnerships – the legal status
- Away day – planning for the future
- Going for gold

INHERITANCE TAX – RELEVANT BUT OVERLOOKED

Currently (2008/09), inheritance tax (IHT) is payable where a person's wealth is in excess of £312,000. Basically, IHT is charged on personal wealth together with all or a proportion of lifetime gifts made in the seven years preceding death. However, on deaths after 9 October 2007, a spouse's unused portion of the nil-rate band is available, against the second spouse's estate, although the maximum is two nil-rate bands per person irrespective of the number of marriages entered into. The full rate of tax is 40%, but this is reduced on a sliding scale for gifts made between three and seven years before death.

IHT is becoming increasingly relevant to GPs following increased earnings and improved pensions under the new contract. The vast majority of GPs live in owner-occupied dwellings valued far in excess of £312,000. Add to this their savings, life assurance policies and their stake in the surgery net assets and it is easy to see why IHT can no longer be ignored. The following need to be considered:

- the value of your assets (now and in the future)
- your financial security
- your family's needs.

Before rushing into a financial plan, GPs should first consider the exemptions and reliefs that are currently available, which are broadly as follows.

- Each individual is entitled to a £312,000 nil-rate band.
- Most transfers between spouses are exempt, but remember that when an estate is left in its entirety to a spouse it will be added to his or her estate and when he or she dies, although for deaths occurring after 9 October 2007 the remaining portion of a spouse's nil-rate band can be offset against the second spouse's estate.
- A GP's stake in the medical practice (including the surgery premises) will normally attract 100% business property relief provided that the assets are disclosed as partnership assets (on the practice sheet). Assets held personally outside the partnership balance sheet may attract only 50% business property relief. Furthermore this relief could be put under jeopardy depending on the wording contained in a partnership deed. If the deed makes it an *obligation* on existing partners to buy out a deceased partner's share, as opposed to an option, then the relief could be withdrawn. This is why most solicitors draft the clause as an option rather than an obligation.
- The first £3,000 of lifetime transfers in any tax year plus any unused for the previous tax year. Remember that a spouse will have a similar exemption.
- Gifts of up to but not exceeding £250 per annum to any number of persons.
- Gifts made out of income that form part of normal expenditure and do not reduce the standard of living.
- Gifts in consideration of marriage per person to bride and/or groom of up to £5,000 by a parent, £2,500 by a grandparent, or £1,000 by any other person.
- Gifts to charities, whether made during lifetime or on death.

These exemptions and reliefs are all very well but are unlikely to solve the problem in its entirety. Other issues need to be considered such as:

- What degree of control would you want your children to have over any assets you may transfer to them?
- How much would your spouse need if you were to die first?

Subject to the above answers, there are some opportunities to reduce the IHT liability as follows.

- Transfers of assets between spouses are exempt from IHT, but other lifetime gifts may be more tax efficient.
- Lifetime gifts are potentially exempt from IHT, and there is no limit on such transfers, so this is an excellent way of transferring assets that you do not need to keep in your estate. It may be advisable to cover substantial gifts by insurance against death within seven years.
- Trusts let you transfer assets out of your estate for IHT purposes, but enable trustees to exercise some degree of control over the capital or income (and you can be a trustee). There may be an IHT charge, but this would be at 20%, and then only if the transfer is over £312,000 per person.
- Life assurance policies (unless designed to cover IHT liabilities) should be assigned during your lifetime so that the proceeds do not form part of your estate on death. The most common assignees are spouses, family members and trusts.

So what is the first step? Successful IHT planning has to be a team effort and GPs are advised to enlist the help of professional advisors (probably their accountant) with a view to the making of a will, which will ensure that:

- your assets are distributed in accordance with your wishes
- you choose the executors and trustees who will carry out your wishes
- you plan the distribution in a tax-efficient manner
- you can provide for gifts to children and others which fall within the nil-rate band for IHT
- you can skip a generation if you wish and provide for grandchildren, which will avoid at least one charge to IHT that would otherwise have arisen on the death of their parent(s)
- you can create flexibility by setting up a Discretionary Will Trust, thus leaving the decisions to trustees nominated by you who can be guided by a (non-binding) letter of wishes.

Given the wealth of GPs and rising property values, IHT is no longer a tax that can be ignored. Proper planning is essential and it is never too early to seek appropriate advice and get the house in order.

(Note: the nil-rate band for 2009/10 is £325,000 and for 2010/11 it is £350,000.)

GP-OWNED PHARMACIES – AN OPPORTUNITY?

There are those, including the Dispensing Doctors Association, pharmacists and the GPC, who have a vested interest in preventing more GP practices successfully applying to dispense. However, the view of the Office of Fair Trading was that the control of entry regulations for pharmacy should be completely abandoned.

The government responded to this opinion by agreeing in principle but limiting the deregulation to large shopping developments, pharmacies with very long opening hours and one-stop healthcare centres. By way of further limitation, the Department of Health (DoH) has inserted a 'necessary or desirable' clause.

So how does this affect GPs? Given that it is government policy to have 'one-stop' health premises, then GPs developing their own pharmacies on site will probably meet the 'desirable' criteria. Provided that there is no pharmacy close by, say within 100 metres, then the 'necessary' criteria will probably also be met. In this way, an application will most likely be granted. Of course, this does not preclude GPs buying up existing pharmacies if they can identify those available for sale.

On the downside, GPs may not own pharmacies, but this can be overcome by GPs setting up limited companies to undertake the task. On the upside, the superintendent pharmacist alone is responsible for the running of the pharmacy under the code of conduct of the Pharmaceutical Society, which means that the GP's time commitment is minimal. In fact, a GP's responsibility will be restricted to general guidance, the observing of company law and the decision as to what to do with the profits.

There are further advantages of considering on-site pharmacies, as follows.
- The ability to provide complete primary care.
- Further use of the site by developing other one-stop services such as health visitors, dentists, opticians and social workers. In other words, the pharmacy can be part of a full health centre development undertaken by GPs.
- Possible availability of improvement grants to extend the premises for the 'one-stop' purpose in accordance with the NHS plan.
- An in-house pharmacy will attract almost 100% of prescription items. No wonder GPs have found no difficulty in finding pharmacists to rent space in a new surgery development – there are so many sources of income.
- Some enhanced services work can be farmed out to the pharmacy.

Of course there are costs involved, but the expense of those who have undertaken the development suggests that the income far outweighs the costs and hassle involved. Even those GPs who have bought out existing pharmacies in the main street have hitherto reported financial success. As GPs hold their away days and set out their future strategy, it is worth considering whether it would be opportune to own a pharmacy.

STAFF PAY – DICTATED BY BUSINESS DECISIONS?

Before the new contract, practices tended to replace staff on a like-for-like basis with one eye always on the level of reimbursement. However, since 1 April 2004 the staff reimbursement has been absorbed in the global lump sum (via minimum practice income guarantee, MPIG) or the personal medical services (PMS) contract sum, which, in a nutshell, means that the practice now has the freedom to decide the exact composition of the workforce. Given this freedom of choice there are a number of points that practices need to take on board to effect a new approach.

- An optimum staff-mix will generate a higher income.
- The right staff must be in place to help practices achieve the maximum quality points.
- Work out the look of your staff skill-mix as if you were starting up a new practice.
- Compare your current staff-mix with the ideal and plan how to achieve the latter.
- When considering staff skill-mix examine whether there are any jobs that would be better done by someone else in the team, ensure that your staff feel valued and part of the team, check that staff are being fully utilised and that you have no surplus members, assess the staff training needs and deal with underperformers.
- Evaluate the skills required to carry out each role in the practice.

Having considered the above points, practices must plan ahead with courage and a will to change, as finding the optimum staff-mix under the new contract will require a fresh approach. The planning will involve:

- Bringing in new or complementary skills as posts become vacant
- Using disciplinary procedures to deal with underperforming staff
- Allocating protected time for monitoring quality points
- Reviewing practice nurse workload
- Assigning data management to a computer-literate team member
- Allocating key roles to specific individuals who have the appropriate skills.

Recently a report on NHS pay entitled *Agenda for Change* (AFC) has been introduced into the arena. One of the key objectives of AFC is to evaluate and redefine the roles within the NHS, which will help practices seeking the optimum staff-mix. However, adopting AFC is not compulsory as GPs are independent contractors to the NHS – the decision will depend on the local labour market, i.e. ability to recruit and retain staff. Whatever practices choose, they should remember that staff contracts must correctly reflect their terms and conditions, and that any proposed change to the method of calculating staff salaries should be undertaken only after consultation with an employment solicitor.

This brings us on to another issue that is exercising the minds of GPs, and that is performance-related pay. As GPs now have the freedom to decide on the composition of the workforce, it is not surprising that they now recognise that bonus systems enable staff to share in the GPs' rewards and allow practices to keep pay rises under control. Such schemes are never easy to set up, and in fact should not be considered at all unless there is an identifiable benefit to the practice. The matters that need to be considered when setting up a bonus scheme are broadly as follows.

- The qualifying team members.
- Rewards can be money based or leave based.
- A money reward can be graded or 'all or nothing'.
- The objectives of each staff member, which should be relevant, achievable, measureable, specific and possibly time-based.

Overall, bonus schemes should be simple, as complicated formulae can upset the team and defeat the purpose at the outset.

Over time, AISMA members will be monitoring staff efficiency by surveying practice accounts to determine the percentage of staff cost to practice income. In this way we will be able to produce local and national averages, which will provide practices with a measure as to their return on staff investment. In the meantime, as a helpful guide, this is how staff should be paid under AFC.

	AFC pay scales	*2007/08*
Band 1	Telephonist, medical records clerk	£12,182–13,253
Band 2	Healthcare assistant, receptionist	£12,577–15,523
Band 3	Healthcare assistant (higher level), secretary	£14,437–17,257
Band 4	General office manager, administration team leader	£16,853–20,261
Band 5	Less experienced practice nurses (E grade)	£19,683–25,424
Band 6	Majority of practice nurses (F and G grades), practice manager (group practice)	£23,458–31,779
Band 7	Nurse practitioners, senior practice nurses (H grades)	£28,313–37,326
Band 8	Nurse consultants employed by PCT or PCO	£36,112–43,335
Range A		

SURGERY PREMISES – AN INTERESTING TALE

We recently came across an interesting scenario that may be of interest to readers. The facts of the matter are as follows.

In 1989, a four-partnered practice entered into a cost rent development equally at a total cost of £180,000. The practice negotiated a partnership loan of £180,000 with their bankers for a term of 25 years. However, because three of the partners wished to have endowment-linked mortgages and the senior partner wished to have a repayment mortgage, the £180,000 was divided into two loans, one for £45,000 and the other for £135,000. The former loan was secured by means of life assurance on the life of the senior partner, whereas the endowment policies in respect of the latter loan were assigned to the practice bankers. The life assurance and endowment policy premiums were paid personally by the individual partners.

As an aside, it is worth noting that all partners were legally, jointly and severally liable for the entire practice loans of £180,000 irrespective of the differing repayment methods and the belief that they were responsible only for their share of the practice loans at any point in time. This is relevant in that the endowment loan of £135,000 was a dormant loan, with only interest being paid whereas the £45,000 loan was being repaid over time. In other words, the senior partner always believed his liability was less than it was on a strictly legal basis. Fortunately, this did not become an issue.

On 31 March 2001, the senior partner (Dr A) retired but retained his owner-ship of the surgery premises. At that time the practice accounts disclosed the property capital as follows.

	Dr A £	Dr B £	Dr C £	Dr D £	Total £
Cost of premises	45,000	45,000	45,000	45,000	180,000
Loan	(28,000)	(45,000)	(45,000)	(45,000)	(163,000)
Equity	17,000	–	–	–	17,000

Following his retirement, Dr A left his 'equity' in the practice, but continued to receive from the practice his share of the cost rent less the loan repayments attributable to the repayment mortgage. In the meantime, Dr's B, C and D con-tinued in practice and replaced Dr A with a salaried GP who was not interested in surgery ownership.

Recognising that the premises were no longer suitable for practising medicine in 2004, the partners negotiate a PFI scheme, which is duly accepted. Accordingly, they place the existing surgery premises for sale, even though they are aware that being in a deprived area they may face a negative equity situation.

At 31 March 2004 the property capital accounts are disclosed in the accounts as follows.

	Dr A £	Dr B £	Dr C £	Dr D £	Total £
Cost of premises	45,000	45,000	45,000	45,000	180,000
Loan	(25,000)	(45,000)	(45,000)	(45,000)	(160,000)
Equity	20,000	–	–	–	20,000

In April 2004, the practice received the best offer yet for the premises which amounted to £120,000, and they were advised by their agents to accept it, which they duly did. At the same time they asked for the surrender values of the endowment policies, and were told that this amounted to approximately £11,000 each, i.e. £33,000.

Given the situation, we could restate the property capital accounts as follows.

	Dr A £	Dr B £	Dr C £	Dr D £	Total £
Value of premises	30,000	30,000	30,000	30,000	120,000
Endowment policies	–	11,000	11,000	11,000	33,000
Loans	(25,000)	(45,000)	(45,000)	(45,000)	(160,000)
Positive/(negative) equity	5,000	(4,000)	(4,000)	(4,000)	(7,000)

Thus, we are in a negative equity situation. The PCT were approached under the new property framework and they were prepared to provide a grant to meet the mortgage deficit costs. However, the PCT insisted that the shortfall was only £7,000 and not £40,000 because of the existence of the endowment policies. Drs B, C and D were in a quandary – do they retain their endowment policies and take over personal loans of £15,000 each, or do they surrender the endowment policies and take over personal loans of £4,000 each? In the event, the partners decided to cut their losses and surrender the endowment policies. Thus, of the £160,000 owed to the bank, £120,000 was cleared from the proceeds of the surgery premises, £33,000 was cleared from the surrender of the endowment policies, and consequently £7,000 remained outstanding. However, Dr A had to be paid out his equity of £5,000 and so the loan became £12,000, being £4,000 each to Drs B, C and D, which was duly paid off by way of PCT grant.

At least all of the above gives you some idea of how the mathematics work. However, it does also lead us to make some general comments as follows.

- Depending on the level of cost rent, it seems that Dr A may have been better off than the other partners.
- Endowment policies obtain most of their value towards the end of the term of policy. Unless GPs believe they are a permanent fixture in the practice for the foreseeable future, they *may* not be the most appropriate form of investment.
- Endowment policies are difficult to value at any point in time – one can normally only use surrender values or the price they can be sold at in the open market.

Varying types of loan in one practice in respect of one premises is difficult to account for fairly and could also cause legal problems in a dispute. Joint and several liability exists unless the loans are personal.

The moral of the story is to seek professional help at the outset and be absolutely clear in what you are trying to achieve and how it will be accounted for along the way. Remember also that the use of investment vehicles involves risk – investments can go up or down as many have found out to their cost in recent years.

WHERE IS THE GOODWILL?

In an alleged attempt to encourage alternative providers to invest in primary care and to increase patient choice, the government has relaxed the rules on the sale of goodwill, which have existed since 1948. But does this mean anything tangible to the GP? We make it absolutely clear that it is still illegal for GPs to buy or sell the goodwill of the essential services provided by an NHS practice.

The effect of new regulations is that certain categories of providers will be outside the scope of the previous ban, as follows:

- existing providers of out-of-hours, additional and enhanced services who do not hold a list of registered patients
- existing GP cooperatives providing the same services where they do not hold a list of registered patients
- new providers entering into the field who do not hold registered lists, including separate legal entities such as limited companies formed by existing GMS or PMS practitioners who only provide out-of-hours, additional or enhanced services.

Consequently, apart from the provision of out-of-hours, additional or enhanced services by cooperatives and commercial organisations, GPs will only be able to take advantage of the new rules if the services are provided by entities which are legally distinct from the practice providing essential services. This, of course, can include a separate partnership in which the identities of some of the partners are different from those in the original partnership. A single-handed practitioner would have to form a limited company to provide out-of-hours services, additional services or enhanced services.

To take the drastic and burdensome route of a separate legal entity, there would have to be some financial advantage to be gained – in particular, some goodwill to generate and ultimately sell. A purchaser has to be attracted to make an investment into a venture that is no more than likely to make the investor a substantial return. The price paid will be totally commensurate with the likely return. So far as concerns additional services and enhanced services, the primary care organisations (PCOs) have a direct interest in keeping profits low – so where is the return? With out-of-hours services there is already considerable competition between commercial providers and cooperatives, and GP practices are unlikely to obtain the prices necessary to generate the sort of profits that will attract a buyer.

On top of all this, contractors cannot subcontract any of their rights or duties under a contract in relation to the provision of essential services to former practices or any entity in which the contractor is involved. Furthermore, if a contractor forms an entity designed to avoid the goodwill restriction, the PCO can terminate the GMS or PMS contract. So where does all this leave us? Will alternative providers actually be encouraged to enter the enhanced services market? If GPs themselves attempt to set up a separate legal entity to provide enhanced services, what impact will this have on the future recruitment of partners who may not be able to afford the entry price?

There is one further but significant problem. A business that is entirely dependent on one person, probably the skilled founder and proprietor, can rarely generate goodwill. This means that the business may not be attractive at all if the owner is no longer there, as the goodwill disappears with the owner. This is particularly true where the business has built up its reputation on the skill of a single person, and where the reputation disintegrates on the retirement of that person. Thus individuals forming entities to deal with medico-legal reports, minor surgery laser clinics, etc., are unlikely to realise any significant goodwill at all when they retire. The trick is to build up an organisation of several skilled individuals where the reputation is the entity itself and not a particular individual, so that the business will continue and remain profitable even after the retirement of the leader.

The other trick is to choose a specialism that does not attract much competition but satisfies the needs of the population. Then, and only then, will GPs generate goodwill. Thus we can envisage organisations setting up minor surgery centres or the like where the organisations could be GPs themselves or completely alternative providers. Maybe the supermarket chains will introduce flu vaccinations or private clinics.

It remains to be seen whether the lifting of the existing provisions will encourage alternative providers to invest in primary care and thereby increase patient choice. What seems clear at this stage is that it will be rare indeed for GPs to 'make a killing' on the sale of goodwill. Perhaps the most likely benefit is for GPs to get together with commercial organisations to provide specialist enhanced services that are not only highly skilled but also in great demand – no doubt commercial advertising will finally dictate what the future will bring.

FROM MANAGER TO PARTNER?

GMS2 introduced a practice management competency framework that imposes further responsibilities on practice managers in the area of quality data collection and financial management. Furthermore, PCOs enter into an agreement for medical services with practices and no longer with individual GPs. As all partners will sign the contract with the PCO, for the first time non-clinicians have the opportunity to contract directly with the PCO in the capacity of a partner, and this will be legally recognised under the contract. This all gives GPs the opportunity to consider the career paths of their practice managers, and in particular whether they believe that it would be a reward to the manager's contribution by giving them an incentive to maximise practice earnings. There are, of course, many implications of making a practice manager a partner, both accounting and legal, and GPs are advised to take full advice before embarking on such a route.

For those GPs who are reluctant to go into full partnership with a practice manager, as an alternative they may consider the salaried partnership option.

This is essentially a prestige issue that affords promotion to the position in name only, as the manager remains as an employee and continues to be taxed as such (Schedule E). However, part of the salary package can be paid by way of bonus linked to practice profitability, should this be desirable. In these circumstances, the practice manager will retain their employment rights with none of the risks or responsibilities associated with unlimited liability partnerships. However, it would be appropriate to draw up a proper salaried partnership contract which should state clearly the master-servant relationship, hours of work, the paid leave for holidays, sickness arrangements, maternity and paternity rights, place of work, and their inability to hire and fire staff at will. In this way, the status of the practice manager will be clear and unconfused. Thus, a salaried partner would not be able to sign the PCO contract as such. Finally, if a salaried partner's name should appear on the practice letterhead, the equity partners need to indemnify the salaried partner against an action from those who advance credit to the practice in the belief that the individual is a full partner.

For those GPs who wish to consider promoting the practice manager to full partnership, there are a number of issues that have to be taken on board, not least of which is the consideration of whether such an appointment may hinder the recruitment of clinical partners in the future.

One major issue is a partnership deed. Either a separate partnership agreement can be drawn up with the practice manager, or the existing deed can be amended to a multidisciplinary document. Whichever is the case, the document should not contain any clinical duties but be specific about relationships with the GPs. It may be appropriate for clinical partners to give a non-clinical partner an indemnity in respect of third-party claims, although it should be borne in mind that if the GPs have no money with which to indemnify the practice manager, then the practice manager will have to pay from their own pocket. Voting rights given to a practice manager should be restricted to non-clinical issues. The deed should also limit a practice manager's responsibilities to areas such as finance, human resources, premises, etc.

At the present time only unlimited liability partnerships are eligible to sign up to a PCO contract. Thus, the practice manager as an incoming partner will assume unlimited liability for the debts and liabilities of the practice alongside the GP partners, because they will also be an owner of the practice. This applies even if the practice manager is guaranteed a base salary and the GP partners have agreed to compensate the practice manager for any practice issues under the terms of an indemnity. The indemnity is worthless if the GPs have no money.

Under GMS2, insurance will become an issue. Patients will be registered with the practice and not with individual GPs. Hitherto, GPs secure 100% indemnity insurance for clinical claims, but practice managers do not have the benefit of such cover. GPs must therefore consider taking out comprehensive practice insurance, as well as individual clinical cover, to protect themselves, the practice as a whole and any non-clinical partners.

As a full partner, the practice manager is deemed to be self-employed, even if there is a base salary attached to the arrangement. As such, the practice manager will be giving up employment rights such as automatic maternity and paternity leave, and in particular compensation that employees may receive in the event of any redundancy or dismissal case. Of course, such protection may be re-instated in the partnership deed.

Buying into surgery premises could also be an issue. If a practice manager is to be included, then the mortgagee or landlord must be approached to gain their consent. GP partners will require proof of a practice manager's financial standing before allowing them to buy into the premises and partnership, as any threat of a potential bankruptcy could result in the mortgagee calling in the loan or the landlord terminating the surgery lease.

Finally, we turn to tax and pensions. The change from employee to self-employed means that instead of tax and NIC being paid under the PAYE system as the responsibility of the employer, it becomes the responsibility of the individual. The practice is advised to seek advice from its accountants as to the ramifications of the change of status. So far as concerns pensions, most practice managers will currently be members of the NHS Pension Scheme for staff, which has certain benefits. We understand that the DoH has confirmed that non-clinical partners will be included in the NHS Pension Scheme, although the mechanics are as yet unclear. Before changing the status of the practice manager, the practice must approach the Pensions Agency to determine exactly what needs to be done to protect all pension rights. At the present time, it is unclear whether non-clinician partners will benefit from the dynamised pension factor.

As with most issues there are pros and cons in making a practice manager a partner. The issue is certainly not simple, and what the above demonstrates is that practices must seek specialist accountancy and legal advice before embarking on what must be considered a significant change in the way medical services are provided in the UK.

ANOTHER TAX TIME BOMB WAITING TO EXPLODE?

All GPs who are self-employed partners in a practice that has an accounting year-end date of anything other than 31 March have to be aware of the potential tax liability that awaits them when they retire or leave the practice for any other reason. This liability arises because of the 'overlap' of accounting periods on which the GP is assessed for tax. This can best be explained by considering a real-life example as follows.

Dr A joined a four-partnered practice on 1 September 2006 on a fixed share of income of £47,250 for the first 12 months, after which he became a parity partner. The accounting year end of the practice is 30 June. Thus far his earnings have been:

1 September 2006 to 30 June 2007 (10 months, 10/12 of £47,250)	£39,375
1 July 2007 to 30 June 2008 (1 year)	£90,000

The important issue is how these earnings fall to be taxed in the relevant fiscal years. The situation is as follows.

Fiscal year

2006/07, based on period 1 September 2006 to 5 April 2007, being £39,375 × 7/10 =	27,563	
2007/08, based on first 12 months in practice, being 1 September 2006 to 30 June 2007 =	39,375	
1 July 2007 to 31 August 2007 (£90,000 × 2/12) =	15,000	81,938
2008/09, based on year to 30 June 2008 =		90,000
Total earnings assessed to tax over three fiscal years =		£171,938

It can be seen that there are two overlapping periods in the above calculations which enable us to calculate the 'overlap' relief to carry forward to retirement or leaving the practice as follows.

1 September 2006 to 5 April 2007	27,563
1 July 2007 to 31 August 2007	15,000
	£42,563

This overlap relief therefore represents nine months of earnings which have effectively been assessed to tax twice in the above calculation, for which relief is given at a later date. So what is the problem? The problem is Dr A has deferred tax to be paid back at a later date. The potential liability is calculated as follows.

Nine months of current earnings, say £90,000 × 9/12 =	67,500
Nine months of overlap relief carried forward =	42,563
	£24,937
Potential future tax liability at 40% =	£9,975

Thus, in less than two years Dr A has created a tax time bomb for the future of £9,975, and it is essential he is aware of this situation to enable him to plan his future career path.

Indeed, many commentators claim that to avoid this future problem it is better to pay tax on an actual basis and thus have an accounting year end of 31 March or 5 April. But is this really correct? What actually happens is that Dr A would have paid an extra £9,975 tax in 2006/07, 2007/08 and 2008/09, in order to save it at a later date. In other words, by having the 30 June year end, Dr A has deferred £9,975 in tax payments to pay at some future unspecified date. To prove the point, let us look at the earnings that would have been assessed to tax had the year end been 31 March.

2006/07, based on period 1 September 2006 to 31 March 2007, being 7/10 × £39,375 =	27,563
2007/08, based on year to 31 March 2008, being 5/12 × £47,250 plus 7/12 of £90,000, i.e. £19,687 plus £52,500 =	72,187

2008/09, based on year to 31 March 2009, say =	97,125
Total earnings assessed to tax over three fiscal years =	£196,875
With a June year end we already know (from above) that the total earnings assessed to tax over the same three fiscal years was	£171,938
Excess of March year end over June year end	£24,937
Tax at 40%	£9,975

It is clear that a rush to change the accounting date is not appropriate – the question is: do GPs want to pay the tax now or defer until later?

If the deferment of tax route is taken, it is essential that GPs know the extent of their 'overlap' tax time bomb in order to plan for the future.

Please make sure that your accountant keeps you advised of this potential future liability so that you don't get a shock when you leave the practice or retire.

CAPITAL ACCOUNTS MADE EASY

One of the most common problems accountants face is the understanding among GPs of how capital or current accounts operate. Both terms mean just about the same thing, but whichever is used, GPs seem to switch off because it is 'jargon' to them – goodness knows, they ought to be used to it!

Let's keep it simple by considering a hypothetical example. Drs Y and Z set up a brand-new practice on 1 January 2008. They purchase surgery premises for £100,000 and spend a further £25,000 on furniture, fixtures, fittings and equipment. Each doctor puts £15,000 of their own money into a practice bank account, and they take out a property loan of £110,000 to finance much of the above capital expenditure. Thus, on day one, the balance sheet of partnership/ practice is as follows.

Partners' capital accounts		
Dr Y	15,000	
Dr Z	15,000	
	£30,000	
Represented by:		
Tangible fixed assets		
Surgery premises	100,000	
Furniture, fixtures, fittings and equipment	25,000	
	125,000	
Less: Bank loan	110,000	
		15,000
Practice bank account		15,000
Total Net Assets		£30,000

The partners decide to pool all income and expenditure and share the net earnings of the practice equally. The question is: what happens to the capital accounts of Drs Y and Z over the passage of time? Let us assume that the practice buys a computer for £5,000 for which no reimbursement is received. In the above example, the tangible fixed assets rise to £130,000, but the practice bank account falls to £10,000. In total, the balance sheet value remains at £30,000, so that the capital accounts must also be £30,000. If the surgery premises are revalued either upwards or downwards, this will have a corresponding effect on the partners' capital accounts. It follows that the reality of the situation is the partners' capital accounts will only change over time depending on the earnings of the practice compared to each partner's drawings.

Let us now assume that in the first year ended 31 December 2008, the income less expenses of the practice amounts to £140,000, which is split equally between the partners. The partners have also agreed to meet their own tax liabilities personally. The records of the practice disclose that the partners have taken the following amounts in drawings.

	Dr Y	Dr Z	Total
Monthly drawings	48,000	48,000	96,000
Superannuation contributions	3,498	3,498	6,996
Class 2 NIC contributions	102	102	204
Quarterly special drawings	16,000	12,000	28,000
	£67,600	£63,600	£131,200

Let us also assume that there is no stock of drugs at 31 December 2008 and that all income has been received (i.e. no debtors) and all expenditure incurred has been paid (i.e. no creditors). Also, the fixtures, fittings, furniture and equipment have been depreciated by £6,000 (20%) to arrive at the net earning of £140,000.

In a nutshell, the formula that always applies to partners' capital accounts is as follows.

Capital account at beginning of period
Add: Share of practice earnings
Less: Drawings
Equals: Capital account at end of period

Thus, the capital accounts of Drs Y and Z at 31 December 2008 will be as follows.

	Dr Y	Dr Z	Total
At 1 January 2008	15,000	15,000	30,000
Earnings year to 31 December 2008	70,000	70,000	140,000
	85,000	85,000	170,000
Less: Drawings (above)	(67,600)	(63,600)	(131,200)
At 31 December 2008	£17,400	£21,400	£38,800

The total of £38,800 will be a 'mirror image' of the net assets of the practice, which will be disclosed as follows.

Tangible fixed assets		
Surgery premises	100,000	
Furniture, fixtures, fittings and equipment	24,000	
	124,000	
Less: Bank loan (after £2,000 capital repaid)	108,000	
		16,000
Practice bank account		22,800
		£38,800

We are now able to define what a partners' capital or current account actually is – it represents the partners' share of the net assets (or worth) of the practice, or the amount of capital introduced by a partner plus earnings not drawn to date. Capital introduced plus undrawn profits (subject to revaluations) will always equal a partner's share of the net assets of the practice.

STAMP DUTY LAND TAX (SDLT) AND MEDICAL PARTNERSHIPS

The SDLT regime as it relates to certain transactions concerning partnerships is set out in the Finance Act 2004, which introduced a new Schedule 15 to the Finance Act 2003. The complexity of the new regime is indeed the subject of controversy and concern in the legal profession. By way of general overview, we set out below a brief summary of the new SDLT rules.

The new rules apply to transactions after 22 July 2004. Before then the old stamp duty rules (i.e. not SDLT) applied to transactions between partners.

First, this new regime does not affect transactions whereby land is acquired from third parties by the partnership, e.g. partners acquiring land for development. Here the normal SDLT rules set out in the Finance Act 2003 apply.

The new regime in Schedule 15 affects general partnerships, limited partnerships and also note that it applies to limited liability partnerships. It concerns three situations:

1 transfer of land into a partnership by a partner
2 transfer of an interest in a partnership
3 transfer of land out of a partnership to a partner.

1. Transfer of land into a partnership by a partner

SDLT is charged on a proportion of the market value of the land transferred plus a proportion of any actual consideration paid for the transfer. The definition of the two proportions is in fact different, and involves the careful application of the formula and definitions set out in the Schedule. This is commented on further in section 3 below.

The aim of the rules is the principle of transparency – the land is regarded as jointly owned by partners and a charge is sought to the extent that there is a change in that joint ownership.

2. Transfer of an interest in a partnership

This is the section (in Paragraphs 14 and 36 of Schedule 15) which has caused most controversy.

Schedule 15 defines a 'partnership interest' as those rights which include participation in profits, right to distribution of partnership assets on a dissolution and liability for a partnership debt.

There is a transfer of an interest in a partnership where 'arrangements' are entered into whereby either (a) a partner transfers the whole or part of his interest as a partner to another person (who may or may not already be a partner) or (b) a person becomes a partner and an existing partner reduces his interest in the partnership or ceases to be a partner.

For the transfer of an interest in a partnership to be chargeable to SDLT the relevant partnership property must include an interest in land and there must be consideration for the transfer.

Relevant partnership property is any land held as partnership property immediately after the transfer. This includes property held by one of the partners and used for the partnership business. But the definition excludes market rent leases. Market rent leases are essentially defined as those without a premium and are either less than five years' term or if longer than five years that there are rent reviews at market rent at least every five years.

There is consideration for the transfer in situation (a) if money or money's worth is given by the person acquiring and in situation (b) if there is withdrawal of money or money's worth from the partnership.

However SDLT is charged on the 'chargeable consideration', which is a proportion of the market value of the relevant partnership property. In the case of a person joining the partnership this proportion is their partnership share after the transaction.

Where the person acquiring the interest was already a partner, i.e. increasing their share, then the proportion of market value of the relevant partnership property is the difference between their partnership share before and after the transaction.

Each partner is entitled to £150,000 nil rate of chargeable consideration. Partnership transactions are only notifiable to the extent that the relevant value exceeds the threshold, so many transactions may not require notification.

What has led to some of the controversy is that the partnership share is the partners share in the income profits of the partnership, rather than the capital account.

Notably the admission of a new partner who contributes cash only with no corresponding withdrawal by an existing partner should not itself give rise to a charge.

It is also notable that unless there are arrangements whereby the funding of the retirement of a partner is dependent on the introduction of a new partner, there is no transaction under Paragraph 36, therefore no charge under Paragraph 14 of Schedule 15. Arrangements would extend to the positions where the withdrawal of money or money's worth by the retiring partner could only proceed with the introduction of money or money's worth by the new partner, or the guaranteeing of a loan by the partners to enable repayment to the retiring partner or some other arrangements, whereby funding which was not then available to allow the retiring partner to withdraw his capital was put in place, including funding of the withdrawal over a period.

A series of helpful examples of how the rules work in practice are set out in the *Inland Revenue Practice Manual*.

3. Transfer of land out of a partnership to a GP partner

Transfers of land out of partnerships are essentially treated in a similar way to incoming transfers, again involving the application of the formula set out in the Schedule. The charge applies where partnership property (comprising land and including leases) is transferred from a partnership to a partner or former partner or to a person connected with such partner or former partner. The broad principle is to measure the relevant chargeable proportion of the property and apply this percentage to market value, where relevant, and actual consideration.

The charge is on a *proportion* (first) of the market value of the land transferred or the Net Present Value of the lease plus a *proportion* (second) of any other actual payment (cash, property in exchange or debt assumed) for the transfer. The first proportion means the proportion of the land *not* retained or treated as retained by the transferee. The second proportion means the proportion of the land retained or treated as retained by the transferee.

Further detail is provided in the Schedule as to method of calculation of the percentage of ownership retained or treated as retained by the transferee, which is referred to as the sum of the lower proportions. Where there are several joint owners, who may be partners or connected with partners, the calculation involves calculating proportions for each relevant owner which take account of connectedness with partners, and adding the resulting lower proportions. In the case of transfers out of a partnership, the calculation also seeks to take account of the profit sharing during the period that the partnership owned the property.

Conclusion

The summary provides some further insight into the complexities of the SDLT regime for partnerships. Application of the SDLT regime to a particular partnership transaction would need bespoke consideration.

DR SOLICITORS
www.drsolicitors.com
Tel 01483 511 555
Fax 0870 762 0245

Editor's note:
We are grateful to DR Solicitors of London for contributing the above.

BUYING IN TO A PRACTICE

It now must be clear to most of us that the recruitment of GPs is very much geared to the concept of supply and demand. The new contract has created a situation where salaried GPs are now striving to become equity partners once again, whereas for financial reasons equity partners would prefer to recruit salaried GPs. Because of surgery ownership and the practice 'bidding' process it is likely that there will be a significant increase in the number of equity partners over the next few years. It is therefore appropriate to consider methods of 'buying in' for incoming equity partners.

Set out below is an extract from the AISMA model accounts Upside Medical Practice at 31 March 2006. For the sake of illustration, let us assume that Dr Prodit retired on 31 March 2006, at which time Dr Preventit agreed to become a property owner, and Dr Lancit was appointed an equity partner on immediate full parity and also agreed to become a property owner. The partners obtained a professional valuation of the property at 31 March 2006 which amounted to £300,000.

	Note	2006	2005
PARTNERS' FUNDS			
PROPERTY CAPITAL ACCOUNTS	13	85,100	61,700
PARTNERS' CURRENT ACCOUNTS	14	52,922	56,733
		£138,022	£118,433
EMPLOYMENT OF FUNDS			
TANGIBLE FIXED ASSETS	15	264,801	256,463
LOANS	16	(174,900)	(188,300)
		89,901	68,163
CURRENT ASSETS			
Stock of drugs		5,016	4,918
Debtors and prepayments		108,732	106,250
Cash at bank and in hand		92,397	83,912
		206,145	195,080
CURRENT LIABILITIES			
Creditors and accrued charges		39,129	37,475
Provision for income tax	17	118,895	107,335
		158,024	144,810
NET CURRENT ASSETS		48,121	50,270
		£138,022	£118,433

13 Property capital accounts

	Dr A Prodit	Dr I Pokit	Dr S Treatit	Dr M Curit	Dr A Preventit	Total
At 1 April 2005	15,425	15,425	15,425	15,425	–	61,700
Transferred from partners' current accounts (Note 14)	5,850	5,850	5,850	5,850	–	23,400
At 31 March 2006	£21,275	£21,275	£21,275	£21,275	£–	£85,100

Represented by:

Freehold property (Note 15)	260,000
Less: loans (Note 16)	(174,900)
	£85,100

14 Partners' current accounts

	Dr A Prodit	Dr I Pokit	Dr S Treatit	Dr M Curit	Dr A Preventit	Total
At 1 April 2005	10,763	10,602	11,425	12,228	11,715	56,733
Net income for the year (page 3)	130,551	131,885	127,276	128,819	126,249	644,780
	141,314	142,487	138,701	141,047	137,964	701,513
Monthly drawings	61,200	60,000	63,600	63,600	66,000	314,400
Equalisation	6,763	6,602	7,425	8,228	7,715	36,733
Seniority drawn	10,841	5,129	4,663	4,663	600	25,896
Class 2 NI	111	111	111	111	111	555
Superannuation:						
– standard paid	6,600	6,600	6,600	6,600	6,600	33,000
– standard provided	493	1,034	711	330	169	2,737
– on other NHS income	496	–	–	334	347	1,177
PAYE/NI on hospital appointments	379	–	–	115	132	626
Taxation – paid 2005/06	17,000	17,400	16,350	16,625	16,200	83,575
– provided 2005/06	23,980	24,550	23,370	23,815	23,180	118,895
Private income	350	8,225	4,125	5,225	8,880	26,805
Personal expenses	(3,624)	(3,191)	(3,988)	(4,435)	(3,970)	(19,208)
Transferred to property capital accounts (note 13)	5,850	5,850	5,850	5,850	–	23,400
	130,439	132,310	128,817	131,061	125,964	648,591
At 31 March 2006	£10,875	£10,177	£9,884	£9,986	£12,000	£52,922

Let us consider some of the options available:

- Dealing first with the partners' current accounts, Dr Prodit needs to draw £10,875 from the practice, which could be afforded by the practice. So far as concerns Dr Lancit he needs to introduce approximately £10,000 to be on a par with the other partners. He can either achieve this by an immediate injection of £10,000 into the practice by way of, say, personal loan, or he could restrict his drawings by £400 per month for his first 25 months to catch up over a period of time. All practices are different, but the restriction of drawings method is often favoured by incoming partners.

- So far as concerns the surgery premises, both Dr Preventit and Dr Lancit could take out personal loans for £25,020 each, introduce these funds into the practice, Dr Prodit would withdraw £31,275, and the other continuing partners would withdraw £6,255 each. This is best illustrated by plotting the movement in the property capital accounts as follows:

	Dr A Prodit	Dr I Pokit	Dr S Treatit	Dr M Curit	Dr A Preventit	Dr D Lancit	Total
At 31 March 2006	21,275	21,275	21,275	21,275	–	–	85,100
Revaluation	10,000	10,000	10,000	10,000	–	–	40,000
	31,275	31,275	31,275	31,275	–	–	125,100
Introduce	–	–	–	–	25,020	25,020	50,040
Withdraw	(31,275)	(6,255)	(6,255)	(6,255)	–	–	(50,040)
At 1 April 2006	–	25,020	25,020	25,020	25,020	25,020	125,100

- The equity of £125,100 above is represented by the value of the property £300,000 less the loan of £174,900. Thus, Dr Preventit and Dr Lancit would assume responsibility for their share of the loan, and Dr Prodit would be released from any responsibility towards the property loan. Dr Preventit and Dr Lancit will obtain personal tax relief on the interest incurred on their personal loans.
- The disposal of his property share is a chargeable event for capital gains tax purposes as far as concerns Dr Prodit (he is disposing of a 25% interest). Likewise there could be capital gains tax implications for Dr Pokit, Dr Treatit and Dr Curit, who are each disposing of 5% of their share in the property, although this is unlikely to be significant.
- Dr Preventit and Dr Lancit may, of course, be unhappy about raising personal loans of £25,020 each. In these circumstances there may be an alternative approach available with the help of the practice lenders. It may be possible for the practice to 'top up' the loan of £174,900 to the valuation of £300,000 so that the equity in the surgery premises becomes exactly zero. This route provides the practice with £125,100 cash which is distributed equally to Dr Prodit, Dr Pokit, Dr Treatit and Dr Curit, being £31,275 each. The tax treatment is exactly the same as above – raising additional finance is not a chargeable event for capital gains tax purposes. The benefit of this approach is that Dr Prodit is paid

out, Dr Pokit, Dr Treatit and Dr Curit release their own equity long before they otherwise might have anticipated, and Dr Preventit and Dr Lancit do not have to raise personal loans. Thus, Dr Preventit and Dr Lancit can buy in by merely accepting their 20% share each of the new practice loan of £300,000. The downside of this approach is that there is no longer any equity in the property and the new loan has to be serviced out of current practice earnings, particularly cost or notional rent.

The moral of the story is that there are a number of ways of achieving a buy-in and proper advice is essential at an early stage. In this example, Dr Lancit can achieve a buy-in without raising any personal finance at all, by a combination of loan top up and restricted drawings for a period of time.

EQUALISATION OF PARTNERSHIP SHARES

We make no apology for returning to the subject of partners' capital or current accounts as many GPs still believe that they are 'paper' entries under the province of the accountant and have no real meaning. The truth of the matter is that they are of fundamental importance in that at any point in time they represent a partner's share of the value of the practice. Accordingly, it is good practice to ensure that the balances on the capital or current accounts are as close as possible to the relevant sharing ratios. Otherwise, there is a strong argument to support the charging of interest on capital or current accounts so that no one partner is penalised for an exceptionally high balance which is effectively financing the partnership for no tangible return. Let us deal with the issue by using a simple but hypothetical example.

Let us assume that we have a dispensing practice of four partners who own the surgery premises equally but share profits (and losses) in the following ratio:

Dr A	21.875%
Dr B	28.125%
Dr C	21.875%
Dr D	28.125%

At 31 March 2007, the surgery is valued at £800,000 and there is a loan outstanding of £745,000. The property capital accounts correctly state each partner's share in the equity of £55,000 in the premises at £13,750. Thus the property capital accounts represent each partner's share in the surgery premises at any point in time. It therefore follows that the partners' current accounts represent each partner's share in all of the remaining assets and liabilities of the practice at any point in time. At 31 March 2007 the remaining assets and liabilities were as follows:

Fixed assets	£	£
Fixtures, furniture, fittings, computers and equipment		32,782
Current assets		
Stock of drugs	16,603	
Debtors and prepayments (amounts owing to the practice)	148,119	
Cash at bank and in hand	121,116	
	285,838	
Current liabilities		
Creditors and accrued charges (amounts owed by the practice)	98,386	
Provision for income tax 2006/07	87,703	
	186,089	
Net current assets		99,749
Value of the practice (excluding surgery premises)		£132,531

The partners' current accounts which represent the value of the practice (excluding surgery premises) were disclosed as follows:

	£	£
Dr A	43,167	
Dr B	36,016	
Dr C	40,082	
Dr D	13,266	
		132,531

It now becomes clear that the above amounts do not reflect the profit-sharing ratios stated above, and that the 'ownership' of the practice value is not as intended. In particular, Dr A might ask why he or she is financing more of the net assets of the practice than the others without compensation in the form of interest.

Many GPs ask how these balances get so much out of line. There are several reasons for this, the most common being as follows.
- One partner incurs tax at source on an outside appointment.
- If the practice pays the tax liabilities of the partners, these liabilities may vary greatly for a variety of reasons.
- Since 1 April 2004, the individual partners' superannuation contributions, both employers and employees, may vary significantly, particularly if one partner is engaged in substantial out-of-hours activities.
- The regular drawings may be incorrectly calculated by not properly taking account of prior shares and charges, and possibly seniority.
- Some partners may have taken out added-years contracts which are not properly reflected in the regular drawings.
- Changes in sessions undertaken during the year.

Once partners' current accounts get 'out of line', corrective action needs to be taken, probably by way of equalisation drawings, which, in the above example, was effected as follows. Dr D was a new partner who had not 'bought' into the practice when joining. It was agreed, with the concurrence of Dr D, that this be corrected, and he arranged to take out a personal loan of £15,000 to inject into the practice. The practice manager further confirmed that there was £32,531 cash in the bank account that was not needed by the practice for working capital and could therefore be drawn by the partners. In total, we have therefore £47,531 to play with to effect an equalisation of the partners' current accounts.

The method of equalisation is to recognise the start and end points. The start point must be the balances on current accounts at 31 March 2007 which are set out above. The end point must be the revised partners' current accounts in profit-sharing ratio, which, after paying out the surplus cash will be as follows:

	£	£
Dr A	21,875	
Dr B	28,125	
Dr C	21,875	
Dr D	28,125	
		100,000

Thus, to get from the start point to the end point the transactions must be as follows:

	Dr A	Dr B	Dr C	Dr D	Total
	£	£	£	£	£
Balances a 31 March 2007	43,167	36,016	40,082	13,266	132,531
Capital introduced by Dr D	–	–	–	15,000	15,000
	43,167	36,016	40,082	28,266	147,531
Equalisation drawings	(21,292)	(7,891)	(18,207)	(141)	(47,531)
Revised current account balances	21,875	28,125	21,875	28,125	100,000

The partners now own the value of the practice in profit-sharing ratio. To maintain the equilibrium, such an equalisation should take place annually, and practices need to ensure they save to enable the transaction to be carried out.

Partners' current accounts represent real value and are therefore not a 'paper' entry dreamed up by accountants. In fact, they form the basis of a payout to a retiring partner, so that once equalised, Dr A would be entitled to £21,875 plus his equity in the surgery premises on leaving the practice. Again, it should be pointed out that the balances on partners' current accounts represent *all* the assets and liabilities of the practice, not just the bank balance, which is why partners will never be able to draw down to nil. They need to leave behind sufficient to finance the practice, such as the furniture or the stock of drugs in the fridge and monies earned not yet received, often referred to as 'working capital'.

PRACTICE-BASED COMMISSIONING – AN OVERVIEW

With the encouragement of the government, commercial providers are waiting in the wings to take over aspects of primary care – in fact it has already started albeit at a slow pace at the present time. But are GPs going to sit back and allow, say, supermarkets to provide a one-stop shop so that a patient's care needs can be dealt with at the same time as the weekly shopping? In truth, GP practices hold all the cards as they already have the patients and are being invited to commission for services. While GP practices have a good track record on rising to challenges (such as QOF), their record of working together is sketchy. There is, however, no doubt that the challenges will be difficult to meet by conventional practices, and collaboration will be necessary to survive in the new market for healthcare.

Government policy is to increase competitiveness within the NHS in the hope of achieving value for money, or cost savings in the eyes of the cynic. The following factors may well have influenced their thinking.

- QOF payouts have far exceeded expectations.
- Access targets are showing no signs of improving.
- Investment in PMS has shown little solid evidence of benefit.
- PCTs have perhaps failed to deliver a cost-effective transfer of services into primary care.

Thus, the new contractual options such as specialist personal medical services (SPMS) or alternative provider medical services (APMS) were introduced.

To deal with this new threat or opportunity, GP practices are beginning to discover the advantages of working collaboratively to share clinical and management expertise and the burden of financial risk. Local medical committees (LMCs) are now advising practices to meet the challenges of competition and commissioning by:

- collaborating
- forming larger groups or partnerships
- establishing GP cooperatives
- creating PBC consortia
- working in partnership with the PCT.

In this way, GP practices can provide or host such services as community nursing, health visiting, therapy and community hospital services rather than leave such services to acute hospital trusts, community NHS trusts, private companies or out-of-hours providers. However, commissioning services, managing budgets, and providing services are not easy matters as they bring with them regulations, responsibilities and risks that require expert financial and human resource management. Given the need to be involved in competitive tendering, working collaboratively would seem to be the only answer.

It seems to us that GP practices have little choice but to get involved, and now it is the only game in town. A creditable consortium of GPs must surely be the best option because of their trustworthiness and concern for patient care – commercial organisations are more accountable to their owners! The alternative is unthinkable – there is a real threat that GPs could lose their independence from the NHS and have no choice but to become employees of a commercial APMS organisation; some already are!

Given that collaboration is the answer, we are sometimes asked what is the most appropriate structure to operate under. There is no right or wrong answer as it will depend upon what the grouping agree to do together, although hopefully they will agree to work more formally as a PBC cluster. For a change, tax and finance are unlikely to be the main drivers. Far more important will be mutual respect and accountability. Consequently, the main driver of the structure will be 'convenience'.

However, by way of summary, the following might be the possible models to consider:

- **Federation** – this is rather like a joint venture whereby practices jointly tender for services. The federation employs some staff, for example specialist nurses and managers, to work between practices. In these circumstances practices keep their separate identities but each contributes to strategic management tasks, perhaps on a pounds per patient formula, for commissioning and provider functions. The net income of the federation might be distributed to practices on the basis of volume and work done.
- **Partnership** – practices may choose to merge to become bigger partnerships. Beware that big partnerships do not suit everyone, as the personalities have to fit.
- **Limited liability partnership** – an umbrella organisation like a federation but more formal, and could be a provider organisation, using the APMS of SPMS model. This would allow it to tender for contracts to deliver more care outside hospitals, using expertise and special interests available across the patch, or buying it in as required, including from consultants.
- **Limited liability companies** – more formal still, but it depends on how far the 'grouping' want to go. Companies can be set up to run other practices. This requires proper governance structures and registration with the Healthcare Commission, and demands management expertise. This route could be used to set up pharmacies, day care units, and even consultant-delivered services, but should really be contemplated only if the intention is to take on the big firms.
- **Specialist PMS schemes** – SPMS allows any NHS trust employee or approved medical or dental performer to set up an NHS company to provide specialist services to patients without responsibility for essential

medical services. PMS and GMS practices can group together to form a specialist PMS scheme and provide NHS services across practices, for example, community hospital services, specialist diabetic nurses and community nursing. In such schemes, employed staff can receive NHS pension benefits.

The choice of structure is geared to how ambitious or otherwise the group want to be. Finance issues come later. One thing is certain: the future of the medical profession is at stake. Surely it is better to be independent in a group with peers rather than be swallowed by a large NHS trust or commercial provider.

PARTNERSHIPS – THE LEGAL STATUS

Since 1 April 2004, corporate bodies have been able to negotiate with PCTs to obtain a contract for the provision of medical services, yet medical practices have thus far been reluctant to change their structure from partnerships to limited companies. This is due to a number of valid financial reasons, such as the following.

- Loss of the benefit of the NHS Superannuation Scheme.
- For accounting year ends other than 31 March, there would be 'catch up' tax and 'catch up' pension contributions known as the overlap tax and pension time bomb.
- Dividends from limited companies are thus far not pensionable.
- Accounts would be publicly disclosed and in a format not necessarily helpful to the management of a practice.
- The administrative burden of compliance with the Companies Acts.
- The potential tax disadvantages of transferring surgery premises into a limited company.
- Higher professional fees.
- Directors' salaries will attract penal employer's national insurance contributions.

It is therefore unlikely that there would be a 'rush' to incorporate even if the superannuation issue were to change if the Department of Health were so inclined. Accordingly, a reminder of the legal status of partnerships is considered timely.

There is only one major piece of legislation that governs all partnerships, including those in general practice – the Partnership Act 1890. This act is unusual in parts in that certain provisions (concerning partners' relations to one another) may be varied by agreement between the partners. Only in the absence of any agreement on these issues will the act's provisions apply. The act is divided into four main parts as follows.

- Definition of partnership.
- Relations with non-partners (the outside world).

- Relations of partners between themselves.
- Dissolution and its consequences.

Definition of partnership

The first clause in the act sets down that: 'Partnership is the relation which subsists between persons carrying on a business in common with a view of profit'.

The meaning of business in common is important because partners can only be held liable for debts in relation to this 'business'. For GPs this usually means the provision of general medical services to a list of patients.

Obligations to the outside world

The act imposes a joint and several liability on each partner for partnership debts incurred while he or she is a partner. This liability *cannot* be waived by agreement. For business purposes every partner is an agent of the partnership and anything done in the ordinary course of the business binds the partnership and the other partners. Such a liability may extend to a debt incurred by a person acting, or apparently acting, on behalf of the partnership, if the creditor is unaware that the person does not have the authority of the partners.

The joint-liability principle includes the possibility that any partner may be sued individually, for example by a patient, and thereby be forced to settle a claim in full. (He or she may then have grounds to sue the other partners for redress.) In some cases a court may require that all the partners be joined in an action. It is also possible that a patient dissatisfied by one partner can sue the whole partnership, hence the vital necessity of all partners having defence body cover. Innocent partners cannot be held liable for *crimes* committed by a partner, but they may be held liable for any civil damages incurred.

Relation of partners between themselves

The rights and obligations of partners to one another are subject to agreement between themselves. In the *absence* of any agreement the following will apply.
- All assets acquired by the partnership become partnership property.
- Partners have a right to an equal share of the capital and profits.
- All partners have the right to take part in the management of the partnership
- No partner may receive 'remuneration' for acting in the partnership business.
- The admission of a new partner requires unanimous consent.
- Only a majority of partners is required to decide on 'ordinary matters'.
- No partner may be expelled unless a power to do so is expressly agreed.
- A partner may dissolve the partnership at any time without notice.

Dissolution and its consequences

Dissolution – the breaking up of a partnership – occurs when the partnership relation terminates, even though the partners may continue to be associated together in a new partnership, or simply to oversee the winding-up of the business. Legally, dissolution will be held to occur because of one of the following:

- by any partner giving notice to the others (subject to agreement)
- by mutual agreement of the partners
- by fraud or misrepresentation
- by a repudiatory breach of the partnership agreement by a partner
- by the death or bankruptcy of any partner (subject to agreement)
- by illegality
- by the order of a court.

Among the grounds on which a court may order dissolution are: when a partner becomes permanently incapable of performing his or her part of the partnership contract (including because of 'unsound mind'); when a partner is in breach of an express or implied term of the partnership agreement; or when the business can only be carried on at a loss.

New partners
It should be noted that the admission of a new partner will as a matter of law constitute a new partnership, therefore his or her liabilities do not extend to those debts incurred before he or she became a partner (and possibly to those after he or she left). However, a new partner *may* be bound by a pre-existing partnership agreement if he or she is aware of it *and* behaves as though it was agreed.

Outgoing partners
Generally, a partner leaving (for whatever reason) will terminate the partnership unless the agreement stipulates that the others will carry on as before.

Written agreement
Because of the problems that may arise, it is recommended that the arrangements between partners should be defined in a written agreement prepared by a solicitor. However, such a document may run to 30 or more pages, so the preparatory work should be broken down into manageable blocks. Set out below are the steps to follow.

Partners should first determine among themselves what financial and other arrangements will apply to the more variable clauses (*see* the 'Important Variables' box below). This will reduce the time spent in arguing in front of a solicitor (who may be paid by the hour).

Next, based on the preliminary discussions, the solicitor should be instructed to prepare a draft agreement. Once this draft is suitably amended it may be signed by all the partners. This may look a simple process but it may take a number of months from start to finish.

Agreements tend to follow a predetermined model and include clauses that are common to all. These 'standard' clauses are either taken from the Partnership

Act or are implied in all partnerships (e.g. to be just and faithful). For the full agreement, *see* the 'Essential Clauses' box. Some of these, like the identifiers, can be written fairly quickly. Others, such as the finance clauses, may already be in operation, as reference to the practice accounts will show. Yet others may be the subject of verbal agreement, such as holiday arrangements.

Each section, identifiers, finance, etc. should be the subject of a separate partnership meeting and a written record kept of what is agreed. Although this process may take some time, it should minimise 'agreement fatigue'. Only when it is completed should partners start instructing a solicitor.

IMPORTANT VARIABLES

Finance	Practice capital
	Practice income – what is included
	Profit shares
	Expenses and their allocation
	Superannuation
Management	Decisions requiring unanimity/majority
	Decision-making process
	Mediation and arbitration
Leave	Holidays
	Incapacity
	Maternity leave
Departure	Expulsion
	Restrictive covenant?

ESSENTIAL CLAUSES

Identifiers	Date of document
	Name and title of practice
	The nature of the business
	List of partners
	Practice address
	Date of commencement and the duration
Finance	The capital
	Practice premises
	Practice income
	Division of receipts – profit shares
	Expenses and their allocation
	Superannuation
	Tax liability
	Accounts
	Banking

Management and decision making	Attention to the affairs of the firm
	Decisions requiring unanimity/majority
	Decision-making process
	Engaging and dismissing staff
	Mediation
	Arbitration
	Defence body membership
Leave arrangements	Holidays
	Incapacity
	Study leave
	Maternity leave
	Paternity leave
	Sabbaticals
Departure	Resignation
	Expulsion
	Lengthy incapacity
	Retirement on age grounds
	Restrictive covenant?

The writer acknowledges the valuable assistance provided by Jim Milligan (a freelance IRO with BMA) in preparing the above article. He can be contacted at <u>www.milliganj. fslife.co.uk</u>.

AWAY DAY – PLANNING FOR THE FUTURE

When formulating the future strategy of the practice, many GPs often find it difficult to get started. Perhaps the best approach is to hold an 'away day', possibly facilitated by a consultant or a specialist practice accountant. The object of the 'away day' is to produce a plan, probably in written form, albeit brief and to the point. To achieve this, practices need an agenda and we set out below a guide which may help the process.

There are a number of prerequisites for any away day, which can broadly be summarised as follows.

- Involve the practice manager either as a facilitator or an integral part of the team.
- Record all major points probably by means of a number of flipcharts.
- All partners must contribute on an equal basis, but be totally honest throughout without being hurtful or unnecessarily aggressive.
- No anecdotes – phrases such as 'in my day' or 'we always used to . . .' are banned.
- No zingers – niggling at each other will not help at all.
- Have plenty of refreshments (but preferably not alcoholic).

The agenda for an 'away day' should centre around six key questions as follows:

Six key questions	Information to consider
1 What do we want to do?	The personal aspirations of the partners regarding healthcare, earnings, general goals and environment.
2 What have we done in the past?	A critical analysis of current and past performance.
3 What must we do well to succeed?	The key success factors.
4 What could we do?	The strengths and weaknesses in terms of resources: skills, staffing, space, finance, etc.
5 What might we do?	The opportunities and threats in a changing environment.
6 What should we do?	The identification and evaluation of a range of options arising from questions (1) to (5).

The above merely *states* the 'bare bones' of the discussion and there may be considerable overlap. To provide more 'flesh on the bone' we set out below the sorts of issues that are likely to be considered under each of the key questions.

Question One: what do we want to do?
- The balance between money and the quality of life.
- How much do you want to earn? How many hours per week do you want to work?
- Organisation chart and lines of authority.
- Partner roles.
- Partnership succession.
- Outside appointments versus NHS.
- Desires to specialise.

Question Two: what have we done in the past?
- How well is the business organised?
- What hours do we currently spend on professional activities?
- How do our earnings compare with national averages?
- How good are we compared to others?

Question Three: what must we do well to succeed?
- The key success factors are normally the essential 'drivers'.
- State-of-the-art premises and information technology systems.
- Structuring the practice properly.
- Delegation of routine tasks.
- Everybody in their correct role?
- Providing the correct services to meet the needs of patients.

Question Four: what could we do?

- What are our strengths and weaknesses?
- Do the partners have the necessary skills?
- Have we got the right staff?
- Are our premises suitable to face the future provision of primary care?
- Do we have the appropriate clinical support in our staffing?
- Are our finances well organised?
- Do we have a good reputation?
- Do we deal appropriately with training needs?
- Do we get on well as a team, meet regularly, and work on the practice as well as in the practice?
- Do we provide the right services?
- Do we have appropriate prescribing and referral patterns?
- Are we happy with our practice profile, quality of healthcare, and list size?

Honesty in considering the practice strengths and weaknesses is crucial.

Whereas question four is rather inward looking, question five considers what is happening outside the practice.

Question Five: what might we do?

- What is currently happening to our profession in terms of NHS direction, government intervention and the provision of healthcare generally?
- Who are our competition and what threats do they pose?
- Might we recruit other healthcare professionals to provide new or improved services?
- Should we train to obtain a specialisation (such as dermatology) which we can 'sell' to the PCT in the form of enhanced services or to our PBC consortium by way of provisioning?
- Can we delegate better to free up our time to take on lucrative outside appointments?
- Might we find land to build a health centre providing a full range of services as owners with selected tenants?
- Are we properly embracing practice-based commissioning and provisioning?
- Have we the resource to 'bid' for other practices?
- Does dispensing provide an opportunity?
- Are there opportunities to obtain income from outside activities?
- Can we achieve more quality points?
- Are there opportunities to reduce costs?

Question Six: what should we do?

Having spent most of the day on questions one to five, it is now time to summarise the practice objectives and philosophy, and list down all the issues the practice is going to address. It is now decision time and all agreed decisions should be written down in the form of a plan. Every decision must state who is responsible for carrying out the task and in what timescale. There should be follow-up meetings to discuss progress, perhaps on a quarterly basis.

To achieve the greatest benefit from an away day, GPs must accept from the outset that a medical practice is a business and success will not be achieved without the:

- right structures
- right roles
- right services
- right technology
- right people
- right premises.

GOING FOR GOLD

AISMA members have been delivering a seminar entitled 'Going for Gold' to various audiences, which looks to protect GP earnings in the future and deals with maximising profits in the new NHS. Readers may be interested in the following synopsis of the presentation.

In order to deal with the future we need to know where we are starting from. According to the NHS Information Centre the average earnings of a GP for 2005/06 was £110,000. However, earnings will vary depending upon whether a GP dispenses and whether he or she operates under GMS or PMS.

For the sake of argument only, and with no supportive evidence whatsoever, let us assume that the following represents average earnings for 2006:

	£
Overall FTE GP	112,500
GMS dispensers	130,000
GMS non-dispensers	102,000
All GMS	107,000
PMS dispensers	145,000
PMS non-dispensers	120,000
All PMS	123,000
All dispensers	135,000
All non-dispensers	109,000

Readers will appreciate that AISMA members review so many practice accounts that several features become clearly apparent in respect of the higher and lower earners. Thus, as a helpful guide to future earnings, here are those features.

Features of high earners

- Stable partnership (low turnover of partners).
- Partners work as a team, trust each other, plan ahead, and meet regularly.
- Top rate databases on patients and treatments.
- Partners have similar philosophies in terms of the dichotomy between money and patient care.
- Proactive rather than reactive teams.
- Good managers of time.
- Well-organised GPs with strong staff teams and good skills mix among them.
- GPs who delegate well to nurses, health visitors, etc.
- GPs who work long hours, have low deputising costs, and high level of non-NHS earnings.
- GPs with very high list sizes (normally single-handed GPs).
- GPs who have the ability to dispense.
- PMS GPs who have taken advantage of growth funding and freed up time to perform more lucrative tasks.
- GPs who are heavily involved with their PCO.
- GPs with the most competent and skilled practice managers and specialist accountants.
- GPs who were early fund holders.

Mark each of the above out of ten

125 or more	= good
100 or more	= average
Less than 100	= poor

Features of low earners – how many apply to you?

- Practices involved in partnership disputes.
- GPs with inadequate resources, such as staff, equipment and space. Such GPs often have the wrong staff mix or have a loyal contingent of staff who have been promoted over the years but do not necessarily have the relevant skills.
- Badly organised practices who typically have an excessive number of patients. Poor internal control systems are a feature of such practices.
- GPs who are bad managers of time.
- GPs who work as individuals and not as a team who gave little or no thought to fund holding or an early entrance into PMS.
- New practices with low list sizes.
- Practices in very deprived areas.
- GPs who value 'time off' way over and above money, who incur very high deputising costs and have a low non-NHS income.
- GPs without the necessary data available on their patients, either through neglect or through poor skills mix among the staff.

Armed with the above, surely practices now have a clue as to what areas they need to concentrate upon to protect future income.

There are of course some key issues to consider in the quest for profitability, which can broadly be summarised as follows:

- Quality points.
- PMS/GMS income per patient (the average is close to £120).
- Calculate your costs as a percentage of total income and compare them to the benchmarks set out in the last edition of this newsletter.
- Consider dispensing which might be an opportunity for practices alone or by way of joint venture.
- Consider level of outside income. (*See* Chapter 7 for the list of 100 ways of obtaining private income.)
- Consider if you are performing sufficient enhanced services – perhaps you have to specialise to become providers.
- Finally, watch your list size – under the new contract money follows the patient!

Having reviewed the above key issues, the next stage is to recognise potential quick-win situations. These can be summarised as follows.

- Bidding for PCT run practices. Remember you need to negotiate £100 to £120 per patient for PMS or GMS contract income.
- Takeover of single handed practitioners – again the £100 to £120 per patient is relevant.
- Get involved in provisioning although this may involve some form of specialisation, such as, by way of example:
  - cardiology
  - elderly
  - diabetes
  - palliative medicine
  - mental health, e.g. substance misuse
  - dermatology
  - musculoskeletal
  - women and children
  - ENT
  - homeless/asylum seekers
  - procedures, e.g. vasectomy, endoscopy.

It will be the locality that determines whether such specialisation is more lucrative than private work.

- Delegate routine tasks to nurses, pharmacists and other health professionals. (GPs are notoriously poor in this art.)
- In a partnership, know where you and your partners stand on the vexed issues of money, patient care and quality of life. If you do not you will all be travelling in different directions.

- Pursue with care lucrative outside appointments, but always consider the opportunity cost. This means you have to measure the benefit of the outside appointment against the cost of what you are giving up. There is *always* a trade off. Beware of the pitfalls of this approach, such as:
  - Ego trip. Flattery, title or status are nice but is a GP a better person for simply filling a vacant post?
  - Escapism. Getting away from the surgery may be great but what is the opportunity cost?
  - Partner resentment. If income is not pooled resentment can occur?
  - Delegation in return. You cannot compress existing surgery work into a shorter time unless you delegate properly. Determine how busy you should be. Letting work mount up is not the way to maximise profit.

As a further consideration in the pursuit of maximising profits, consider how to contain costs. This might be achieved by the following.
- Delegate to practice managers, but do not abdicate; there have been too many horror stories.
- Join buying consortiums, for example, for the purchase of drugs.
- Use internal rather than external locums.
- Shop about for the special deals, but not for your accountancy services.

At the end of the day GPs must realise that medical practice is now a business. The highest earners in the future will be those practices who have the:
- right structures
- right roles
- right services
- right technology
- right people
- right premises.

The future is certainly going to be a challenge.

CHAPTER 17

Financial horror stories

The AISMA quarterly newsletter has recently run a serious of true horror stories that have occurred in medical practice. The series, which readers may find of great interest, is reproduced below.

While the basic stories are absolutely true, names and locations have been fictionalised to protect the innocent and maintain professional conduct. Readers may also be interested to learn that many of the horror stories arise or come to light when a specialist medical accountant takes over from a non-specialist accountant.

HORROR STORY 1

Our true story for this issue relates to a two-partnered practice in the north of England that operated under a PMS contract. After their accounts had been prepared by a non-specialist accountant for the year ended 31 March 2003 and their tax returns completed for the 2002/03 fiscal year, the partners decided to change their accountants to a specialist, in fact an AISMA member. It follows that the first accounts prepared by the new accountants were for the year ended 31 March 2004, which took place in November 2004. During November 2004, the senior partner telephoned the accountants to ask specifically if they could determine why the practice felt short of income – they simply felt that they were earning less than they anticipated but had no idea why. This, of course, is no simple task, but the accountants promised to look in depth into the earnings of the practice.

By the end of November the draft accounts were prepared but there were no obvious anomalies. On stricter examination the accountants noticed that the total PMS contract income had fallen without any obvious explanation. The list size had not fallen and there was no obvious clawback of growth monies. The rest of the accounts seemed consistent with previous years and consequently it was deduced that the problem could possibly relate only to the PMS contract sum. Accordingly, the accountants were drawn into a detailed examination of the

PMS contract. In normal circumstances a PMS contract for the fiscal year ended 31 March in any year is rolled over into the next year with any adjustments in terms of inflationary uplift, lift size, growth, etc. taken into account. However, on this occasion, it was noticed that the normal rollover had not taken place, but instead, for whatever reason, the PCT had set up a new spreadsheet altogether. Accordingly, the accountants took the view that the rollover from 2002/03 to 2003/04 needed to be checked thoroughly to detect any obvious unexplained deviations.

Bingo! The penny dropped! The problem hit the accountants right in the face. In the rollover of the grouping of items which were originally superannuable at 100% under the Old Red Book or old GMS contract, which included baseline seniority, childhood immunisations, pre-school boosters and cervical cytology, the total of £33,700 for these items had in fact been rolled over at £3,370 by absolute clerical error. This had occurred by moving the decimal point one place to the left. On this occasion, no fault can be attributed to the previous accountants as they completed their work at 31 March 2003, although it must be stated that they did not ask to look at the new contract sum at 1 April 2003 to see if anything might have affected the accounts for the year ended 31 March 2003.

By the time the new accountants met up with their client it was already December 2004. Perhaps the surprising aspect of this true story is that neither the practice manager nor either of the partners noticed that the PMS amount had fallen due to the movement of the decimal point. They merely wondered why their income had fallen! The new accountants had the job of explaining to them that their income had fallen due to clerical error for the year to 31 March 2004 on behalf of the PCT, which had continued to present date, i.e. December 2005. The practice was therefore informed by their new accountants that they were owed 21 months of adjustment calculated as follows:

$$£33,700 - £3,370 \times \frac{21}{12} = £53,078$$

The practice was, of course, delighted by the findings but was at a loss as to how to pursue the matter. The accountants therefore undertook to negotiate with the PCT and produced irrefutable evidence as to what had occurred. The practice was pleased to receive a cheque from the PCT amounting to £53,078 on 23 December 2004, just two days before Christmas. The appointment of specialist accountants was already vindicated. As a sequel, the accountants raised an additional charge of £500 plus VAT for the exploratory work, and the practice was again delighted that the PCT met this additional charge in January 2006 by way of interest compensation. A nice happy ending to a *true* story.

However, not all stories have a happy ending. By way of bonus, we now set out a less than happy ending to a true story for this issue alone. Under the days of the old Red Book, an AISMA accountant took over the affairs of a practice from a non-specialist accountant. They noticed that no seniority appeared under

GMS income in the accounts, which appeared odd as the six partners were, to be polite, not spring chickens. On further enquiry it transpired that each of the six partners received seniority personally, direct to their home. It transpired that no entry appeared in the partnership tax computations and no entry appeared on any of the individual partners' personal tax returns.

Without boring the reader with gory details, it was obvious to the specialist accountant that no tax had been paid on seniority payments for a number of years. On this occasion, defeat had to be admitted and each of the partners had to accept tax bills plus interest on six years' worth of seniority, which amounted to a considerable drain on personal finances. This only goes to prove that all true stories do not have a happy ending, but the moral of the tale is to ensure that you have the right professional advisers in place to guide you through the maze of financial complexity.

HORROR STORY 2

This issue involves a situation where one of our members was asked to present their services to a six-partnered urban practice in the north of England who had hitherto used the services of a non-specialist accountant. Our member was successful in securing the appointment, but at the outset the senior partner asked the new accountant if he would review the capital account balances of the partners over the last few years as they had clearly got severely out of line and were nowhere near representing profit-sharing ratio. The senior partner could not understand the differentials at all as he was responsible for calculating the partners' drawings and took great care in ensuring that drawings were equitable.

The new accountant agreed to the above task on the basis of no fee if nothing was found but an agreed 'deal' if something came out of the woodwork. He asked for the practice accounts for the last 10 years up to 31 March 2001. The accountant, true to his promise, undertook the review and found nothing of major importance in the first seven years to 31 March 1998. He then noticed that on 1 April 1998 three of six partners took out added-years contracts which obviously meant that their superannuation contributions were going to be significantly higher than the other three partners. As the partnership shared 'profits' equally it was agreed that the three partners with added-years contracts would pay to the practice the differential in superannuation contributions so that equality would be maintained and the capital accounts would not get unfairly out of balance. The accountant noticed that the balances on partners' capital accounts at 31 March 1998 were quite close and that the imbalance occurred during the three years ended 31 March 2001. The picture was beginning to form and, 'hey presto', a discovery was made.

The accounts were quite well laid out with a reasonable amount of detail. There was a note in the accounts which broke down the NHS income of the practice over various headings. The accountant noticed that included in this note for each of the three years ended 31 March 2001 appeared an item entitled 'added years'. He also noticed that nothing appeared in the partners' accounts for capital introduced by the three partners who had taken out added-years contracts to effectively cancel or offset the charge made to those three partners' capital accounts by way of added years' superannuation deducted at source for these three partners.

Furthermore, because added years was charged to the three partners' capital accounts by way of drawings, the past accountant assumed that this related to 'income' of these partners and consequently included it as part of their private income.

So what was happening here? The situation can broadly be summarised as follows:

- The added years' contributions introduced by the three partners to cancel the charge on them was *not* disclosed as capital introduced but rather disclosed incorrectly as NHS income divided in profit share in error and taxed accordingly.
- The private income of the three partners was erroneously inflated by the added years contributions and taxed accordingly.
- Of the above two items, only the former affected the partners' capital account balances, but both items affected the tax liabilities of the partners.

So what did the new accountant do? First of all, he calculated what adjustments were required to the partners' capital accounts for the three years ended 31 March 2001 had the profit shares been calculated correctly and the added years contributions made by the three partners to the practice been properly disclosed as capital introduced. Lo and behold the balances on the partners' capital accounts ended up very close to the profit-sharing ratio, which was originally intended. The new accountant proposed that these adjustments were made to the capital accounts in the year ended 31 March 2002. But of course this was not the end of the story – there was the thorny issue of taxation to consider.

Accordingly, the new accountant proceeded to redo the income tax computations for 1998/1999, 1999/2000 and 2000/2001. Having completed the exercise, he prepared error and mistake claims for these years and set up a meeting with the local District Inspector of Taxes to go through the claims and agree matters. To cut a long story short, the meeting with the District Inspector of Taxes went well and the Inspector appreciated what had gone wrong and agreed to issue revised tax assessments. The amount of tax overpaid by the partners and due to be refunded with interest was broadly calculated as follows:

Annual added years £4,000 × 3 partners × 3 years × 2 for duplication in practice and private income = £72,000 at 40% tax = £28,800 plus interest.

Finally, the new accountant calculated how the £28,800 was to be divided between the partners and advised the practice accordingly.

The practice was delighted at the outcome. There just remained one final issue to resolve – what was the new accountant's fee for this special one-off exercise? True to his word, the new accountant proposed a 'deal' of a fee of £1,000 plus VAT = £1,175, which was agreed by the practice and duly settled immediately. The final sequel to the story was the new accountant contacting the old accountant to explain what had happened and that the practice was not particularly happy with their work. Accordingly, the previous accountant agreed to meet the fee and VAT of £1,175 and duly reimbursed the practice.

At the end of the day, the practice was happy that matters had been sorted out, its capital accounts were no longer in imbalance, it had received a tax refund of £28,800 plus interest, and this situation had been reached at no cost at all to itself in terms of professional fees. The moral of the story is again clear – medical practices need to engage accountants who know their way around the specialist area of medical finance.

HORROR STORIES 3

On this occasion, instead of relating one horror story in depth we tell a number of short stories. Readers will have noticed that most of the horror stories thus far emanate from one of our members taking over the accountancy work from a non-specialist accountant. However, it would be totally unfair to suggest that all horror stories arise in this way, as we are about to demonstrate.

Our first story concerns a dispensing practice client of an AISMA firm who registered for VAT on 1 April 2006. The situation is that the practice has yet to receive any refunds of VAT. The practice has received two visits from a VAT officer of HMRC. However, the VAT officer is refusing to authorise any repayments of VAT on the basis that in his opinion the practice manager has failed to understand the process. Fortunately, the practice has had the sense to call in their AISMA accountant, who has been able to sort out the situation and is now hopeful that the practice is about to receive a £75,000 refund to bring matters properly up to date.

Our second story concerns an AISMA member taking over the accountancy affairs of a practice from a non-specialist accountant. The situation is best described as 'a can of worms'. In a nutshell the new accountant has discovered that the previous accountant had been using the wrong basis periods for each of the fiscal years running from 1997/98 to 2004/05. Thus, for example, the accounts for the year ended 30 April 1999 form the basis for the fiscal year 1999/2000 and profits should be allocated for 1999/2000 on the basis of what happened in the accounts for the year ended 30 April 1999. However, the previous accountant had allocated the profits in the accounts for the year ended 30 April 2009 on the basis of the profit-sharing ratios prevailing in the fiscal year 1999/2000 – and he had done this for eight successive years. This is truly a nightmare situation and the new AISMA accountant has spent considerable time in preparing calculations to rework all of the tax payments by the partner for the eight years in question.

Having completed the exercise it transpires that the practice as a whole has overpaid tax amounting to £25,000. The problem now is that, of the £25,000, some partners have overpaid tax, some partners have underpaid tax, and some partners are neutral. To make matters worse, new partners have joined the practice, partners have left the practice, and partners have retired so that the constitution of the practice at the end of the eight-year period bears little resemblance to what it was at the beginning. It would be almost impossible to agree all of the revised calculations for the eight-year period with HMRC and then collect the tax and refund the tax to all of the relevant partners, both old and new. But somehow an equitable solution must be found.

While no final decision has been reached, the favourite option is to leave HMRC alone, receive £25,000 from the previous accountant (who has agreed to do same), and allocate the £25,000 to the partners based on the new calculations but slightly favouring those who have overpaid the most tax.

Our third story concerns a continuing client of an AISMA firm. In February 2005 the AISMA member prepared the pension certificates of a three-partnered practice, which were duly signed and forwarded to the PCT. The superannuation shortfall was correctly processed by the PCT and the appropriate deductions were made in March 2006 on the GMS schedule of that month. However, on the same schedule the PCT made a further deduction of £4,800, purporting to be the AVCs of one of the partners, but neither the practice manager nor any of the partners noticed this spurious deduction. Eventually, during the preparation of the accounts for the year ended 30 June 2006, the AISMA firm noticed the deduction and queried how it was to be dealt with in the accounts. On enquiry, it transpired that the partner in question was not contributing to AVCs. On further enquiry with the PCT it transpired that the deduction was indeed a clerical error and they agreed to return the amount forthwith. The moral of the story is absolutely clear – someone in every practice *must* check the monthly PMS or GMS schedule and ensure that *all* items are correct and appropriate. A specialist accountant may ultimately spot the error but it is doubtful whether a non-specialist accountant would.

Our final story yet again concerns a case where a non-specialist accountant was changed for an AISMA member in a six-partner practice. The first accounts prepared by the new accountant were for the year ended 31 December 2006. It should also be noted that the practice manager was a new appointment. During the course of the accounts preparation the AISMA firm noticed that the reimbursement for drugs was considerably less than the value of drugs purchased, suggesting that there may be a problem with forms FP10 which are forwarded to the Prescription Pricing Authority to trigger the reimbursement. On further examination, it was noticed that the monthly drug reimbursement was relatively constant throughout the year, which is odd in itself because it is expected that in one month the reimbursement will be much higher than all other months due to the reimbursement of flu vaccinations. The practice received the enhanced service for flu vaccinations and it became clear that the reimbursement for the cost of the drugs had not been received. On further enquiry it transpired that the new practice manager had not been told to make a claim. She thought that it was an automatic reimbursement from the PCT rather than an FP10 claim to the PPA. However, having been alerted, she decided to discover what had happed in previous years and found that claims for the previous two years had also not been made.

The end result of this story is an FP10 claim for three years' flu vaccinations reimbursement amounting to £40,000. The alarming feature of this story is that this was the third occasion this AISMA firm had come across missed flu vaccination reimbursement claims in the space of three months. The moral of the story is again clear – GP partners can delegate but not abdicate responsibility for the finance function of the practice.

HORROR STORY 4: HOW NOT TO PAY OUT A RETIRING PARTNER!

This true story concerns the retirement of a GP from a five-partnered practice on 31 December 2002. The practice prepared its annual accounts to 30 June each year, operated a dispensary, owned two surgeries and employed a non-specialist accountant. To retain anonymity we will call the GPs Dr A, Dr B, Dr C, Dr D and Dr E, with Dr A being the retiring doctor in question.

On 30 June 2002 the balance sheet of the practice disclosed the following (approximately):

	£	£
Surgery premises (1) at valuation	375,000	
Surgery premises (2) at valuation	75,000	
	450,000	
Less: property loan	(350,000)	
		100,000
Fixtures, furniture, fittings and equipment at book value		20,000
Current assets		
Stock of drugs	45,000	
Debtors and prepayments	75,000	
Cash at bank and in hand	10,000	
	130,000	
Current liabilities		
Creditors and accrued charges	60,000	
Net current assets		70,000
		190,000

Represented by:

Property capital accounts (£20,000 each)	100,000
Partners' current accounts:	
Dr A	20,000
Dr B	19,000
Dr C	17,500
Dr D	18,000
Dr E	15,500
	90,000
	190,000

During the year ended 30 June 2003 the practice appointed a specialist firm of accountants who would prepare the annual accounts for the year to 30 June 2003. However, it was left to the previous accountants to advise on the payout to the retiring Dr A. The first stage of the transaction was undertaken correctly – the practice agreed to pay Dr A £20,000 for his share in the equity of the surgeries and release him from all liabilities connected to the property loans. The practice also agreed to pay him his partner's current account being £20,000 at 30 June 2002, plus an estimate of earnings less drawings from 1 July 2002 to 31 December 2002 (which later proved to be quite accurate).

The situation then went 'belly up'. For some inexplicable reason, the previous accountants advised that Dr A was also entitled to his share of the value of drugs stock and fixtures, fittings and equipment at 31 December 2002 which they calculated at £13,000 (probably £45,000 stock plus £20,000 fixtures, etc. at his share of 20% = £13,000). The practice consequently paid out £53,000 to Dr A.

In September 2003 the new accountants (who are members of AISMA) prepared the practice accounts for the year ended 30 June 2003. These accounts showed that Dr A had overdrawn £13,000 that was due back to the practice. This is because the £13,000 paid to Dr A for stock and fixtures and fittings, etc. was in fact a 'double count' in that these items are already included in his partners' current account as demonstrated by the balance sheet at 30 June 2002 above which of course *balances*. The partners' current accounts are represented by the fixtures and fittings, drug stock, debtors, and bank account, less liabilities – it is therefore clearly a double count if Dr A receives more than his partners' current account for these items.

The practice rightly requested the return of £13,000 from Dr A. Dr A was surprised to receive this request and could not understand why he had been overpaid. He sought advice from the previous accountants and his solicitors and ultimately refused to repay the £13,000. Through his solicitor and accountant, Dr A contended that the practice claim of £13,000 was spurious and that he had correctly been paid out in accordance with the instructions of the previous accountants. On the advice of the new accountants and the practice solicitor, the continuing partners issued a formal demand on Dr A for £13,000. The demand surprisingly was defended with vigour and legal proceedings duly ensued. To this day it remains a mystery why the defendants could not understand what is a relatively simple accounting concept. Nevertheless, substantial costs were incurred by both sides, including the cost of employing barristers! In an attempt to settle the matter, the practice said it were prepared to accept £10,000 in full and final settlement but for reasons best known to himself Dr A appeared to want his day in court.

To cut a long story short, Dr A rightly lost heavily in court, being obliged not only to repay £13,000 to the practice but also the legal costs of both sides, which amounted to a further staggering £40,000. The moral of the story again is to ensure that proper specialist professional advice is sought to deal with the financial arrangements relating to incoming and outgoing partners, and to remember that legal action based on perceived principles is always going to be an extremely costly experience.

HORROR STORY 5

Yet again, this horror story stems from a practice changing accountants from a non-specialist to an AISMA member. This urban practice prepared accounts annually to 31 March and in March 2007 they interviewed the new accountants with a view to taking over matters for 2006/07 as the 2005/06 year in terms of tax, accounts and pension certificates had been completed by the outgoing accountants.

The interview in March 2007 went well for both parties, the meeting being both productive and congenial. The new accountant was particularly impressed with the surgery premises, which were obviously new and state of the art. Upon enquiry, it transpired that the practice had undertaken a major renovation and refurbishment exercise in 2004/05, which was completed in March 2005 at a total cost of £270,000, financed entirely by bank loan. Upon even further enquiry, the practice explained that it had undertaken a similar renovation and refurbishment of its branch surgery which was completed in January 2005 at a total cost of £250,000 and also financed entirely by bank loan. The accountant's only thought on the matter was that due to the incidence of capital allowances it was unlikely that the six partners paid much tax in 2004/05.

The new accountant undertook the usual tasks involved in setting up a new client, which included writing to the outgoing accountant to obtain all of the information necessary to commence acting. The request on this occasion included accounts and all tax returns for 2004/05 and 2005/06. Normally, the request might be for only one year, i.e. the most recent year 2005/06, but the new accountant was alerted to the fact that 2004/05 was a special year because of the property renovations and related capital allowances claims.

The new accountant studied the documents supplied by the outgoing accountants. She discovered the following. First, in the accounts for the year ended 31 March 2005, there appeared two items of additions to freehold property being £270,000 and £250,000 respectively. This was odd in itself because with major refurbishments one would expect much of the above amounts to be allocated to fixtures, furniture and fittings. The tax computations for 2004/05 showed a small capital allowances claim but only in respect of items brought forward from the previous year – there were *no* additions to the capital allowances 'pool' for 2004/05. The situation was no different in 2005/06. More alarming still, the tax liabilities of the partners actually increased in both 2004/05 and 2005/06 following the effects of the new contract.

The new accountant set to work immediately and made due enquiry with the practice as follows:

- Did your accountant discuss capital allowances with you?
  Answer: No.
- Did your accountant ask you to obtain a priced bill of quantities from your architect or quantity surveyor?
  Answer: No.
- Did you receive an improvement grant for any of the works?
  Answer: No.

The new accountant asked the practice to obtain a priced bill of quantities and forward it to her immediately on receipt.

Some weeks later, the new accountant received the priced bill of quantities for both premises which was indeed a very bulky document to scrutinise. Nevertheless, after much hard work she identified the following costs, which would qualify for capital allowances claim at each of the surgery premises:

- Main surgery: £80,000 out of a total cost of £270,000
- Branch surgery: £70,000 out of a total cost of £250,000.

Thus, she had identified a total capital allowances claim of £150,000 which would result in the following claim for income tax purposes in the first five years:

2004/05 first year allowance at 50%	75,000
2005/06 25% writing-down allowance (on reducing-balance basis)	18,750
2006/07 25% writing-down allowance (on reducing-balance basis)	14,062
2007/08 25% writing-down allowance (on reducing-balance basis)	10,547
2008/09 10% writing-down allowance (on reducing-balance basis)	3,164
Total capital allowances claim against income tax for first 5 years	£121,523

Consequently, over a five-year period the above claim generated a tax saving of £49,824 (being £121,523 at 41%). As the 2004/05 and 2005/06 fiscal years had already passed before this exercise was undertaken, the new accountant was able to obtain a tax refund for these two years which amounted to £38,437 (£75,000 + £18,750 at 41%). The practice actually received £40,000 as the amount included an interest supplement.

The practice was naturally delighted, even after it received a fee from the new accountant of £1,500 plus VAT for this special exercise.

One word of caution – the system is changing on 6 April 2008 whereby the claims will be spread over a much longer period.

Index

Page numbers in *italic* refer to tables.